Handbook of
Organ
Transplantation

Handbook of
Organ
Transplantation

Jayshri A Shah MD, DNB, MNAMS, MRCP, CCST (UK)
President, Liver Healthcare and
Wellness Foundation, Mumbai
Consultant Hepatologist, East Kent University Hospitals
NHS Foundation Trust, UK
Member, ZTCC/ROTTO Liver Committee

Sujata Patwardhan MS, MCh (Urology)
Professor and Head
Department of Urology
Seth GS Medical College
KEM Hospital, Mumbai
Secretary, Advisory Committee
ROTTO-SOTTO, KEM Hospital, Mumbai

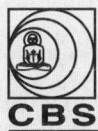

CBS

CBS Publishers & Distributors Pvt Ltd
New Delhi • Bengaluru • Chennai • Kochi • Kolkata • Mumbai
Hyderabad • Jharkhand • Nagpur • Patna • Pune • Uttarakhand

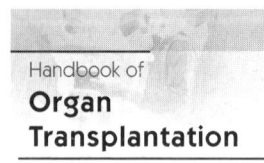

Handbook of
Organ Transplantation

ISBN: 978-93-89017-63-2

Copyright © Authors and Publisher

First Edition: 2020

Reprint: 2021

Published by Satish Kumar Jain and produced by Varun Jain for

CBS Publishers & Distributors Pvt Ltd

4819/XI Prahlad Street, 24 Ansari Road, Daryaganj, New Delhi 110 002, India
Ph: 011-23289259, 23266861, 23266867   Website: www.cbspd.com
Fax: 011-23243014   e-mail: delhi@cbspd.com; cbspubs@airtelmail.in
Corporate Office: 204 FIE, Industrial Area, Patparganj, Delhi 110 092

Ph: 011-4934 4934   Fax: 011-4934 4935   e-mail: publishing@cbspd.com;
                                                publicity@cbspd.com

Branches

• **Bengaluru:** Seema House 2975, 17th Cross, K.R. Road, Banasankari 2nd Stage, Bengaluru 560 070, Karnataka
Ph: +91-80-26771678/79   Fax: +91-80-26771680   e-mail: bangalore@cbspd.com
• **Chennai:** 7, Subbaraya Street, Shenoy Nagar, Chennai 600 030, Tamil Nadu
Ph: +91-44-26680620, 26681266   Fax: +91-44-42032115   e-mail: chennai@cbspd.com
• **Kochi:** 42/1325, 1326, Power House Road, Opp. KSEB, Power House, Ernakulam 682018, Kochi, Kerala
Ph: +91-484-4059061-65   Fax: +91-484-4059065   e-mail: kochi@cbspd.com
• **Kolkata:** No. 6/B, Ground Floor, Rameswar Shaw Road, Kolkata 700014 (West Bengal), India
Ph: +91-33-2289-1126, 2289-1127, 2289-1128   e-mail: kolkata@cbspd.com
• **Mumbai:** PWD Shed, Gala No. 25/26, Ramchandra Bhatt Marg, Next to JJ Hospital, Gate No. 2 Opp. Union Bank of India, Noorbaug, Mumbai 400009, Maharashtra, India
Ph: +91-22-66661880/89   e-mail: mumbai@cbspd.com

Representatives

• **Hyderabad**   0-9885175004   • **Jharkhand**   0-9811541605   • **Nagpur**   0-9421945513
• **Patna**   0-9334159340   • **Pune**   0-9623451994   • **Uttarakhand** 0-9716462459

Printed at India Binding House, Noida, UP, India

Message

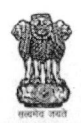

महाराष्ट्र शासन

सूचना का
अधिकार

संचालनालय, वैद्यकीय शिक्षण आणि संशोधन, मुंबई

शासकीय दंत महाविद्यालय व रुग्णालय इमारत चौथा मजला, सेंट जॉर्जेस् रुग्णालय आवार, पी. डीमेलो रोड, फोर्ट, मुंबई- ४०० ००१
दुरध्वनी:+९१-२२-२२६२०३६१-६५/२२६५२२५१/५७/५९. टेलीग्राम: "MEDUCATNSEARCH" फॅक्स:+९१-२२-२२६२०५६२/२२६५२१६८
संकेतस्थळ: http:/www.dmer.org

I am happy to know that Regional-State Organ and Tissue Transplant Organisation [ROTTO-SOTTO], Mumbai, has prepared a manual for transplant coordinators and medical social workers. The theme chosen for the Manual is great and is of interest. It covers various aspects of transplant like ethics, laws, rules and counseling.

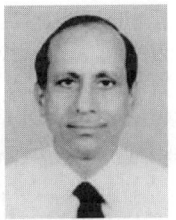

I congratulate the office bearers for providing this ready reckoner for practising transplant coordinators.

I have no doubt that the Manual will provide good source of information to the users.

Pravin H Shingare
Director
Medical Education and Research

Message

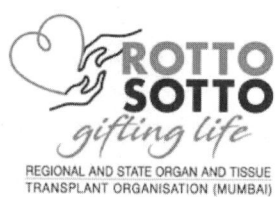

REGIONAL AND STATE ORGAN AND TISSUE
TRANSPLANT ORGANISATION (MUMBAI)

In recent years the Government of India has made great efforts to bridge the chasm between the demand and availability of organs and tissues through its National Organ and Tissue Transplant Programme (NOTP). National, Regional and State Organ and Tissue Transplant Organisations have been set up by the Ministry of Health and Family Welfare to advance this goal, and to establish much needed registries.

The *Handbook of Organ Transplantation* is a valuable resource that furthers this programme. Addressing a critical lacuna in available literature, it targets transplant coordinators who play a vital role in the donation and transplantation of organs and tissues from deceased donors. Offering a one-stop tool for understanding this multidimensional field, it covers trends across the world and national statistics, the anatomy and physiology of donated organs, organ related disease, donation of tissues, applicable laws and regulations, communication and counselling skills, ethical issues and standard operating procedures.

It is a privilege for the Regional-cum-State Organ and Tissue Transplant Organisation (ROTTO-SOTTO), Western Region & Maharashtra State, to support the publication of this Handbook. I am sure that it will benefit not just transplant coordinators but also medical and legal professionals, NGOs, the police and the lay public who form part of the vast network that is essential for a robust organ and tissue transplant programme.

Astrid Lobo Gajiwala
Director, ROTTO-SOTTO
Western Region and Maharashtra State

Message

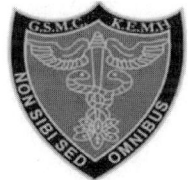

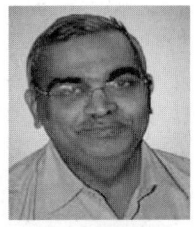

I am very happy to know that ROTTO team is publishing *Handbook of Organ Transplantation*. Congratulations to the team for this excellent work.

Transplant co-ordinators make a lot of difference to success of any transplant program. Our region needs experienced transplant co-ordinators and this manual will facilitate their learning and knowledge of organ transplantation.

This manual provides structured material to understand various aspects of transplant programme including organ functions, diseases that lead to transplantation, laws, regulations and guidelines required for day-to-day working. This manual will complement as a stand-up transplant coordinators material and also as a self-study tool.

I am sure each and every person interested in this field will find this book very useful.

With all best wishes.

Avinash Supe
Director, ME & MH
Dean, Seth GS Medical College
KEM Hospital, Mumbai

Contributors

Abhay Huprikar
Nephrologist, Ruby Hall Clinic and Sahyadri Hospital, Pune
Secretary, ZTCC, Pune

Ameya Sunil Mahajan
Assistant Professor
Rajiv Gandhi Centre for Contemporary Studies

Anirudha K Kulkarni
Manager, Organ Transplant
Jupiter Lifelines Hospitals Ltd., Thane

Ankur Shah
Consultant Hepatobiliary and Liver Transplant Surgeon, Medanta
Institute of Liver Transplant

Anvay Mulay
Consultant Cardiac Surgeon
Fortis Hospital, Mulund, Mumbai

Arati Gokhale
Central Coordinator, Zonal Transplant Coordination Centre, Pune

Arun Kumarraj
Fellow in HPB and Liver Transplant Surgery

Astrid Lobo Gajiwala
Director, ROTTO-SOTTO, KEM Hospital and GS Medical College
Mumbai, and Consultant, Tissue Bank, Tata Memorial Hospital
Mumbai

Balaji Aironi
Associate Professor, Cardiovascular and Thoracic Surgery
KEM Hospital, Mumbai

Bharat Shivdasani
Interventional Cardiologist Coordinator
Department of Cardiology, Jaslok Hospital, Mumbai

Bhavana Shah
MA, PGDHA, MBA in Health Care, Executive Administration and
Sr. Transplant Coordinator, Wockhardt Hospitals
Mumbai

Bhushan Patil
Associate Professor, Urology, KEM Hospital

Darius Mirza
Lead Surgeon–HPB and Transplant Unit
Apollo Hospitals, Navi Mumbai
Professor, HPB Surgery and Transplantation
Queen Elizabeth and Birmingham Children's Hospital, UK

Deepa Usulumarty
Consultant, Nephrologist, Apex Coordination Center

Fysal Kollantavalappil
Associate Consultant, Department of Liver Transplant, Kokilaben
Dhirubhai Ambani Hospital, Mumbai

Ganesh Sanap
Apex SWAP Transplant Registry

Gaurav Mehta
Consultant, Gastroenterology and Hepatology,
Kokilaben Dhirubhai Ambani Hospital, Mumbai

Hunaid Hatimi
Fellow in HPB and Liver Transplant Surgery

Jayshri Shah
Consultant Hepatologist, East Kent University Hospitals, NHS
Foundation Trust, UK
President: Liver Healthcare and Wellness Foundation
Member, ZTCC/ROTTO Liver Committee

Joseph Thomas M
MS, MCh, DNB, FRCS, MNAMS, PGMLE, PGDBE
Professor, Department of Urology, KMC, Manipal
Head, Centre for Bioethics
Manipal Academy of Higher Education

Kamaxi Bhate
Additional Professor, Community Medicine
Seth GS Medical College, KEM Hospital, Mumbai

Meera Suresh
Treasurer, PRO
Snehbandhan Trust, Chembur, Mumbai

MM Bahadur
Director, Department of Nephrology and Transplantation
Jaslok Hospital and Research Center, Mumbai

Nandkishore Kapadia
Director, Cardiac Surgery and
Director, Heart and Lung Transplant Programme
Kokilaben Dhirubhai Ambani Hospital and Research Institute

NK Hase
Professor and Head, Department of Nephrology
Seth GS Medical College and KEM Hospital

Pathik Parikh
MD (Medicine), DM (Gastroenterology)
Apollo Hospitals, Navi Mumbai

Prakash Saindane
Transplant Coordinator, Apollo Hospitals, Navi Mumbai

Prashant Nair
Consultant Cardiologist, Kokilaben Dhirubai Ambani Hospital

Pravin H Shingare
Director, Directorate of Medical Education and Research
Maharashtra

Rahul Pandit
Director, Critical Care, Fortis Hospital, Mulund, Mumbai

Ravi Mohanka
Chief, HPB and Transplant Surgeon, Global Hospital, Mumbai

Rekha Barot
Manager, Transplants and Academics
Kokilaben Dhirubhai Ambani Hospital and Medical Research
Institute

Ruchita Masurkar
Jaslok Hospital and Research Center, Mumbai

Sandip Bhurke
DNB (Nephrology), MD (General Medicine)
Consultant Nephrologist and Kidney Transplant physician
Prabhakar Bhurke Clinic, Andheri [West], Mumbai

Sandeep Sinha
Clinical Coordinator, Fortis Hospital

Santosh B Sorate
Transplant Coordinator
Fortis Hospitals Ltd., Mulund, Mumbai

Saurabh Dhariay
Registrar, Department of Cardiology
Jaslok Hospital and Reasearch Centre, Mumbai

Shanbhudeo S Dalvi
Community Development Officer, KEM Hospital

S Keswani
Plastic Surgeon Medical Director
National Burns Centre

SK Mathur MS, FACS
HPB and Liver Transplantation Surgeon
Vice President & Ag Gen Sec ZTCC, Mumbai
Founder Member, MCFOT & ZTCC
Member, Govt. of MH Committee for Liver Transplantation
Guidelines

Somnath Chattopadhyay
Consultant, HPB and Liver Surgeon, Global Hospital

SP Rai (Col)
Consultant, Pulmonary Medicine
Kokilaben Dhirubhai Ambani Hospital and Research Institute
Mumbai

Sujata Patwardhan
Professor and Head
Department of Urology, Seth GS Medical College, KEM Hospital
Mumbai
Secretary, Advisory Committee, ROTTO-SOTTO, KEM Hospital
Mumbai

Sucheta H Desai
Transplant Coordinator, Hinduja Hospital

Sujata Ashtekar
Consultant, ROTTO, Mumbai
Chairperson, Awareness Activities
ZTCC, Mumbai

Tukaram Jamale
Associate Professor, Department of Nephrology
Seth GS Medical College and KEM Hospital
Mumbai

Urmila Mahajan
Consultant, ROTTO

Viswanath Billa
Associate Professor and Consultant, Nephrology
Director, Apex Kidney Foundation

Vikram Raut
HPB and Liver Transplant Surgeon
Apollo Hospitals
Navi Mumbai

Vinay Kumaran
Liver Transplant HPB Surgery
Kokilaben Dhirubhai Ambani Hospital
Mumbai

Vinita Puri
Professor and Head
Department of Plastic Surgery
Seth GS Medical College and KEM Hospital
Parel, Mumbai

Preface

We are pleased to present *Handbook of Organ Transplantation* which provides a comprehensive overview to all aspects of organ transplantation. The idea to write this book resulted from a conversation, wherein it was discussed that a lot of books have been written on transplantation for clinicians. However, there is very little information for transplant co-ordinators, who are the main pillars playing a key role, acting as liaison among other team members for a successful transplant programme.

The goal of this book is to meet all the requirements, providing a comprehensive overview with practical guidance, covering specifics of each aspect of transplant program administration including evaluation, communication and collaboration with patient, family and clinical staff, ethical issues, government rules and regulations.

The content is based on experience of successful transplant programs as well as suggestions from published literature. We are grateful to the authors who are experts in their respective field. Immense care has been taken by the authors to use simple and lucid language to ensure that the chapters are easily read not only by trained coordinators but also by paramedical staff.

There are various annexures providing valuable information which will help the transplant coordinators in their day-to-day work.

Although this book has been created specifically for use by transplant coordinators, it may have considerable value for transplant administrators and related professionals such as health policy researchers, hospital management staff who are assigned with the task of starting a transplant program. The idea that started as a seed of thought has now blossomed with this book, which hopefully will prove to be a valuable resource to those involved with organ transplantation.

Jayshri A Shah
Sujata Patwardhan

Acknowledgements

We are grateful to all the authors who have spared their precious time for their valuable contribution to facilitate and complement training in the field of transplantation. Particularly grateful to Ms Sujata Ashtekar who has shown immense enthusiasm and worked consistently towards completing this book.

Jayshri A Shah

Sujata Patwardhan

Contents

Section IV: Heart and Lungs

Section V: Cornea, Skin, Hand and Body Donation

Section VI: Communication and Counselling Skills

Section VII: Public Awareness, Motivation and Ethics

Section VIII: Law, Rules, Regulation and Guidelines

Introduction to Organ Donation

Organ Donation East *versus* West

Pathik Parikh, Vikram Raut , Darius Mirza

Over the last 50 years, transplantation has advanced dramatically and with each passing day the number of individuals waiting for a transplant keep on rising exponentially. The gap between the available organs and the numbers needed has been widening. Though this gap is present for all available organs in each of the transplant centers of the world, there is a significant difference between the patterns of donation between different countries. A rough estimate of the need for liver transplant in India is 15000–20000 per year and the current number fulfils only 10% of the requirement. Against a requirement of 1 to 2 lakh kidneys, only about 7000 transplantations are being done annually. This chapter deals with the ethics, policies and pattern of organ donation in the west versus the east.

TYPES OF DECEASED ORGAN DONATIONS

There are three forms of established organ donations which form the source of organs for transplantation; donation after brain death (DBD), donation after cardiac death (DCD) and live related donation. The Uniform Anatomical Gift Act in 1968 prevented donation unless the donor was declared "dead". The concept of brain death was introduced later on, that paved the way for organ donation. Brain death is defined as the irreversible loss of all functions of the brain, including the brainstem. The three essential findings in brain death are coma, absence of brainstem reflexes, and apnea. This is the most established mode of transplant. To counter the scarcity, the other two modes of donations were introduced.

In DCD, the non-heart beating donors, usually with a significant severe brain injury, have suffered circulatory arrest with the heart no longer pumping blood to the organs. In this situation, organ retrieval has to start *as soon as possible* after death has been determined—preferably within the 60 minutes of hypotension (defined as a systolic pressure < 55 mm of Hg). This time period includes an obligatory "stand off" period. This period of hypotension prior to cold preservation comprise the donor warm ischemia period. Most countries utilize only controlled cardiac arrest as suitable organs and the practice is most developed in the United Kingdom, USA, Canada, Australia, Belgium and Holland. Countries like Spain, France and Italy in addition utilize uncontrolled DCD to achieve liver and renal donations. One of the "close" relative donates a portion of the liver or one of the kidneys in live related donation. It initially began for pediatric patients and now used even for adults to adult organ donation.

Regulation and Framework of Deceased Organ Donation: East versus West

In the United States at the time of the first transplants, there was no formal system regulating the procurement process. Donors were identified from within a transplant center, and the organs obtained were transplanted into a patient from that center. Organ procurement organizations (OPOs) are now developed, distinct from a specific transplant center, which allow organ retrieval to be conducted in a more systematic manner. OPOs are established throughout the country and work within their geographical region with one or more designated transplant centers. The first national, computer-based matching system, called the United Network for Organ Sharing (UNOS) was established by OPO. In 1984 the National Organ Transplant Act (NOTA) was passed which led to the establishment of the Organ Procurement and Transplantation Network (OPTN). OPTN is responsible for increasing both the supply of organs for transplantation. OPOs have designated procurement areas known as donor service areas (DSAs). The OPO manages donors within a DSA and is also responsible for care of donors and participate in public education and methods to enhance organ donation.

There is no single system for organ procurement and allocation across the European continent or within the European Union. There are however, different organ exchange organizations for different countries and geographical areas, including the following: Organization National Transplants (ONT) in Spain, NHS Blood & Transplant (NHSBT) for the United Kingdom and Ireland, Euro transplant (Germany, the Netherlands, Belgium, Luxembourg, Austria, Hungary, Slovenia, and Croatia), Scandia transplant (Sweden, Norway, Finland, Denmark, and Iceland), North Italian Transplant Programme (NITP) and Establishment français des Greffes (EfG) in France. All of these work on nearly the same principles. The key players in regulating organ donation in the UK are NHS Blood and Transplant (NHSBT) and the Human Tissue Authority (HTA). Among its responsibilities is to provide a reliable, efficient supply of organs for transplantation. The HTA give approval for organ donations from living

people through an independent assessment process. All potential liver and heart/lung donors in the UK or Republic of Ireland are reported by telephone to the Organ Donation and Transplantation (ODT) Duty Office as soon as the brainstem death tests have been confirmed, or relative's consent has been obtained, or Coroner's consent has been obtained. Each UK center is supplied with donors from their donor zone. The size of that zone and which hospitals are included in it, is dictated by that center's percentage share of all new registrations onto the national elective liver transplant list. For renal allocation, a complex scoring system including the level of donor specific bodies and the level of histocompatibility match are taken into account.

The government of India enacted The Transplantation of Human Organs Act (THOA) in 1994, the first step for regularization of organ donation in India. The aim was to provide for the regulation of removal, storage and transplantation of human organs for therapeutic purposes and for the prevention of commercial dealings in human organs. Over the period of next 10 years the act failed to have significant effect to increase the organ donation as the act implementation was a state subject. THOA was amended in 2008 to improve growth of transplantation in India. THOA defined the terms Appropriate Authority (inspects and grants registration to hospitals for transplantation), Authorization Committee (regulates living donor transplantation), brain stem death, deceased person, donor, recipient, near relative and other such terms to regulate the process of organ donation. It gives a person or his near relative the decision of donation. The donor's own authorization, if it is done before death in presence of two witnesses, is adequate, unless the next of kin has a reason to believe that it was subsequently revoked. THOA outlines the procedure for certification of brain death and recognizes members from the medical board, who are (not members of the transplant team), authorized to certify brain death. The cost of donor management, retrieval, transportation and preservation is not be borne by the donor or their families. THOA prevents hospitals not registered under the act to conduct, the removal, storage or transplantation of any human organ. NTORCs (non-transplant organ retrieval center) are ICU equipped hospitals where organ retrieval alone can be performed once registered with the appropriate authority. Registered non-governmental organizations (NGOs) are roped in to facilitate organ or tissue removal, storage or transplantation; Multi Organ Harvesting Aid Network (MOHAN) foundation is one such NGO.

China still has one of the largest transplant programs in the world and has by far the shortest wait times for organ transplants in the world. Initially, the law allowed the organs to be procured from executed prisoners and that led to transplant tourism but that practice has been condemned worldover and is considered "ethically indefensible". In 2007, the human organ transplant regulation was passed. The Red Cross Society of China has been commissioned by the Ministry of Health to run the organ donation system. It acts as a watchdog to see that organ donation, procurement and allocation within the medical system are done in accordance with the law.

In Korea, the Organ Transplantation Act came into effect in 2000, establishing the Korean Network for Organ Sharing (KONOS) with centralized authority for organ procurement which was revised in August 2002, to introduce an incentive system. If a transplantation hospital formed a Committee for Brain Death Evaluation and a Hospital Organ Procurement Organization, it could receive a kidney from a brain dead-donor as an incentive to foster organ procurement regardless of the KONOS wait list. The Korea Organ Donation Agency (KODA) is the national organ procurement organization established in 2011.

Social and Religious Practices in Deceased Organ Donation: East versus West

The shortage of organs for transplantation makes it important to understand why some oppose organ donation. Religion plays an important role in determining the organ donation practices worldwide. There are different beliefs for different religions about the organ donation. Islam does not allow violation of the human body either in living or dead situation. In 1996, the UK Muslim Law Council issued religious ruling that organ transplantation is entirely in keeping with Islam. However, even in Singapore, where there is a concept of presumed consent, Muslims are exempted from that law. The Christian faith appears to generally endorse transplantation, although there are clearly different nuances in opinion. Transplantation itself was not allowed for Jehovah's witnesses until recently. The Jewish faith places great importance on avoiding any unnecessary interference with the body after death, and the requirement for burial of the complete body (burial within 24 h is the rule). Hindus believe in transmigration of the soul and reincarnation and reports about the use of body parts to benefit others are also deeply embedded. The concept of organ donation is not supported in persons of Chinese ethnic origin due to center Confucianism values, Buddhist, Taoist and other spiritual values. They do not support the thought or organ donation as they associate an intact dead body with respect for ancestors or nature.

The social beliefs also play a role. There are misconceptions that the body of the donor would be mutilated and treated badly, if the person wanted to donate one organ that other organs would also be taken, if a person was involved in an accident the doctors would not save his life if they knew that he was a donor, the relatives have to pay for the expenses for the donation process and finally age fit for donation.

Consenting for Organ Donation: East versus West

In countries like the United States, United Kingdom, Germany, and Netherlands donation is not presumed and either the patients or the family takes the initiative to consent for organ donation. Singapore, Belgium, and Spain have a more aggressive approach of *presumed consent*. Accordingly, the law in these countries permit organ donation by default unless the donor has explicitly opposed it during his lifetime. Some nations like Austria, have considered a third policy; *pure presumed consent* which means that a person must register at a courthouse to express their desire or opposition to be an organ donor.

International Registry in Organ Donation and Transplantation and Indian Transplant Registry

IRODaT (International Registry of Organ Donation and Transplantation) is a database that provides information by country of donation and transplantation activity. 99 countries are reporting to this database. As per the database, in 2015 the percentage per million population (pmp) for US, Canada, Brazil, Argentina, UK, France, Spain, Italy, Croatia, Korea and Japan was 28.5 (n = 9079), 19 (n = 618), 14.10 (2852), 13.75 (593), 20.20 (1311), 25.25 (1627), 39.70, 22.52 (1369), 39 (169), 9.9 (506) and 0.72 (91) respectively. In India the registry (Indian Transplant Registry) came into being with the help of Indian Society of Organ Transplantation (ISOT). The national average of organ donation was 0.26 per million populations in 2012 which became 0.34 in 2014 (Figs 1.1 and 1.2). Until November 2015, 4933 cases of successful voluntary deceased organ donation in total were carried out in China. According to the statistics, the deceased organ donation rate in China currently is about 0.6 pmp.

There are multiple reasons for poor organ donation rates in India. There is lack of awareness and education, inadequate coordination and implementation of policies and even amongst medical professionals the understanding of brain stem death is poor. Finally, what matters is motivation to identify, educate and counsel relatives of potential donors among the intensive care doctors.

Living Donor Transplantation: East versus West

Living donor transplantation is an alternative transplantation option, with lower waiting list mortality and suffering, and equivalent allograft and patient survival than deceased donor transplantation. This has been utilized more frequently in India and South Korea while it is less often utilized in the west. LDLT (Living Donor Liver Transplant) in India is expected to expand to many more centers along with DDLT. As per the database, in 2015 the percentage per million population for west was lower than the east (Fig. 1.3). India is one of the largest centers performing LDLT and a registry is of paramount importance to authenticate and validate the numbers and experience quoted. Most programs are in the private sector and LDLT is the predominant form of liver transplant, a body like the UNOS to overlook all transplants in the country was need of the hour. National Organ and Tissue Transplant Organization (NOTTO) is a similar apex center in India for all activities of coordination and networking for

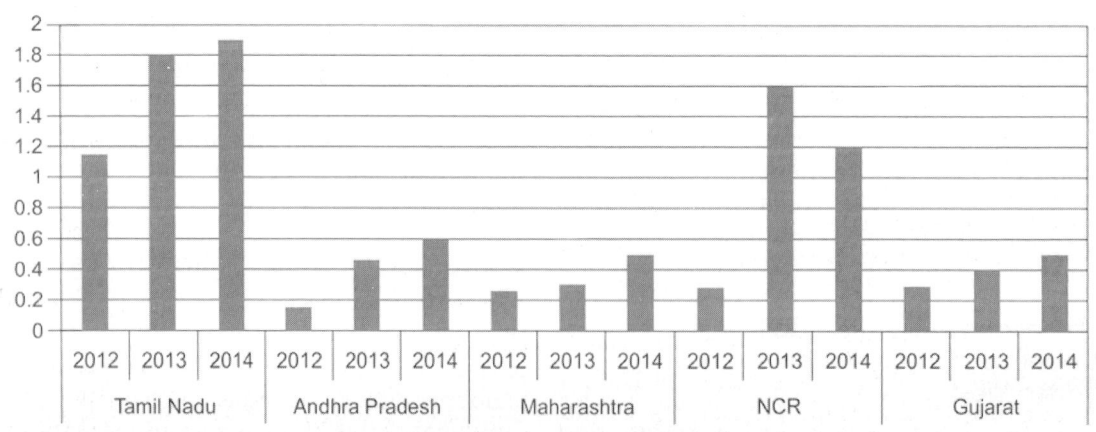

Fig. 1.1: Percentage per million population

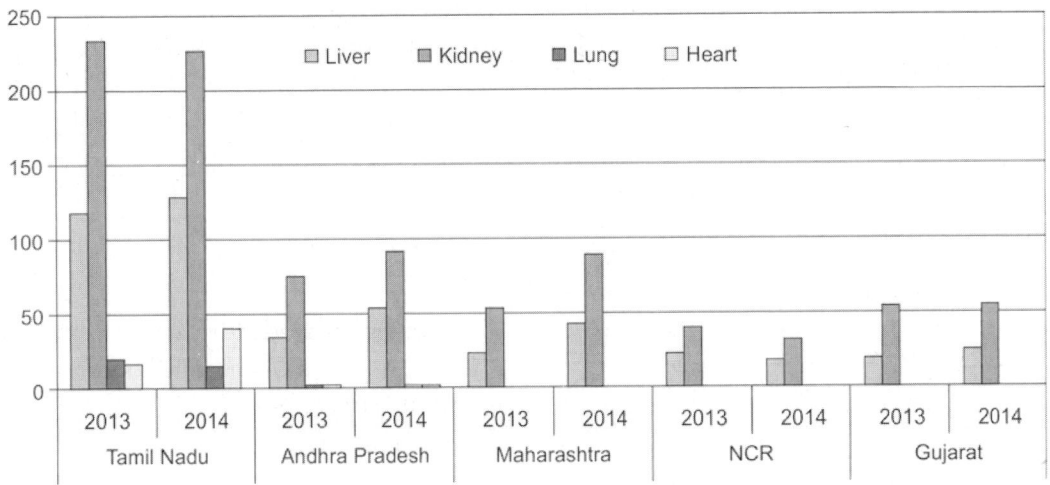

Fig. 1.2: Organ wise distribution in different states

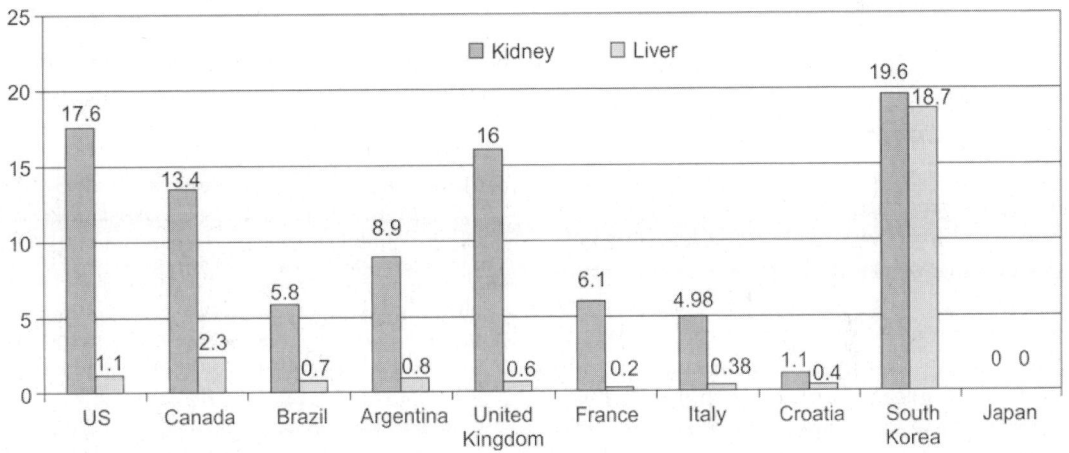

Fig. 1.3: Living related kidney and liver transplant in different countries in the year 2015. It is based on data from IRDOaT. All values are in percentage per million

procurement and distribution of Organs and Tissues and registry of Organs and Tissues Donation and Transplantation in the country. An established registry exists for kidney transplantation and all details can be available on Indian Transplant Registry. There is a specific geographical distribution for liver transplant, LDLT/DDLT divide. North India relies on LDLT predominantly (about 97%) and programs in the south have equal proportions of LDLT and DDLT with some even having a higher proportion of DDLT. According to the data released by China Liver Transplantation Registry (CLTR), over 1,700 cases of LDLT had been completed in mainland China till December 2012, among which no donor death was reported.

Non-heart Beating Donors: East versus West

Non-heart beating donors or donation after cardiac death (DCD) are the answer to meet the increasing demands for organs when DBD organs are not enough and living related donations are not preferred. DCD donations are yet to get a foothold in India though centers have attempted DCD-based transplants. In India, the biggest challenge to DCD donation is lack of clarity in the law, and there is no practice of withdrawal of life support in end of life situation, thereby limiting this mode of donation. There is no notes or representation of organ donation after circulatory arrest in THOA (1994) and in later modifications. Therefore, it can only be used in unanticipated circulatory arrests. South Korea has attempted DCD donations and is still in process to consider it an established mode of donation. From 2010 to 2013, the ratio of DCD liver transplantation to total case numbers in China rose from 1.38% to 26.1%, whereas for kidney, the ratio were 0.59% and 24.6%, respectively. The total number of DCD in China has accumulated to 1564 cases. There were 548 DCD donations in the UK with PMP of 8.40 while in the US 1494 donations (16.5% of all donations) were after cardiac death. DCD organ donations are on the rise in these countries with deceased organ donations remaining static.

Future Directions to Improve Deceased Organ Donation in India

Public awareness and involvement is the key to increase the rate of organ donation. It is necessary to involve society, NGOs, voluntary organization, religious leaders in this movement to encourage people to donate their organs. Success of eye donation campaigns using famous personalities spreading the message is a great example of that. We need to develop awareness strategy for general public keeping in view socio-psycho-cultural belief of society. In Tamil Nadu, who received the best state award in the area of cadaver organ donation, the state government has taken decisive steps to promote organ donation and transplantation, created patient-centric healthcare and green corridors to facilitate organ transfer and donation for the needy persons.

Further Information

1. www.notto.nic.in
2. http://www.irodat.org
3. http://www.mohanfoundation.org
4. http://isot.co.in
5. http://nhsbt.org

Further Reading

1. Narsimhan G, Kota V, Rela M. Liver Trans-plantation in India. Liver Transplantation 2016; 22:1019–24.

2. Shroff S. Current trends in kidney transplantation in India. *Indian Journal of Urology/: IJU/: Journal of the Urological Society of India*. 2016;32(3):173–174. doi:10.4103/0970–1591.185092.

3. Shukla A, Vadeyar H, Rela M, Shah S. Liver Transplantation: East versus West. *Journal of Clinical and Experimental Hepatology*. 2013;3(3): 243–253. doi:10.1016/j.jceh.2013.08.004.

4. Singh NP, Kumar A. Kidney transplantation in India: Challenges and future recommendation. MAMC J Med Sci [serial online] 2016 [cited 2017 Jul 21];2:12–7

5. Soin A S, Thiagarajan S. Liver transplant scene in India. MAMC J Med Sci 2016;2:6–11.

Concept of Brain Death

Rahul Pandit

INTRODUCTION

For understanding what is brain death it is important to know why the concept is being discussed and what is death, is there any legal definition of death? For centuries together the understanding of death has been limited to the death by cardiorespiratory sense, where there is irreversible cessation of circulation and breathing. Previously, death was associated with stoppage of respiration [breathing] after the stethoscope was invented, it was associated with stoppage heart beats. Concept has been so well ingrained that the acceptance of death comes naturally in this situation. In 1951 in USA, death was defined as the 'cessation of life, as a total stoppage of the circulation of the blood ...'

However with the improvement in science and technology, came in the artificial life support systems, defibrillators etc. With this came the realisation that using resuscitation techniques a heart that stopped could be restarted and machines could breathe for the patient, which created a situation where patients with no cerebral blood flow can be maintained artificially for certain period of time. The concept of brain death was thus created by medical progress or, as eloquently stated by Jennett, was 'an artifact of nature resulting from the capacity of medical technology to prolong and distort the process of dying'.

Following this was the *"Sydney Declaration in 1968" in 22nd World Medical Assembly.* The declaration said the following:

- *"...*clinical interest lies not in the state of preservation of isolated cells but in the fate of a person.
- Here the point of death of the different cells and organs is not as important as the *certainty that the process has become irreversible..."* This it was uniformly accepted that if the brain has ceased its functions completely and irreversibly then this state would be called ***BRAIN DEATH.***

This was followed by various criteria been described for diagnosing brain death, like the Harvard Criteria, Minnesota Criteria, etc. Further there was a clear understanding that individually all the tests performed to determine brain function were aimed at brain stem function only, hence the concept of Whole Brain Death including Brain Stem Vs Brain Stem Death was floated. The geographic divide was evident that the British and Commonwealth countries adopted *Brain Stem Death*, whereas America and South America adopted the *Whole Brain Death* concept. Despite varying terminology, the clinical concept of brain death was well established.

It is important to note that the brain death was NOT diagnosed for the purpose of Organ Donation, but for declaring patients dead. More so organ transplantation was just developing and of course brain death brought in the possibility of organ donation.

What does our law say

The Transplantation of Human Organs Act, 1994 (Central Act 42 of 1994).

'Deceased person' means a person in whom permanent disappearance of all evidence of life occurs:

1. By reason of brain stem death or

2. In a cardiopulmonary sense at any time after live birth has taken place.

3. 'Brain stem death' means the stage at which all functions of the brain stem have permanently and irreversibly ceased.

India follows the Brain Stem Death Criteria, it is important we do not mix the two and when we refer it in our communication, especially with the family, we mention it to the family that their loved one is *"Dead"*.

Brain Stem (Fig. 2.1)

Brain Death

Brain death is established by documentation of:

1. Irreversible coma

2. Irreversible loss of brain stem reflexes

3. Cessation of respiratory centre function

The most important aspect of diagnosing brain death is "There is a clear cause of irreversible coma".

This means that brain death is only suspected in patients in whom there is clear cause of irreversible coma established.

Brain Death is Commonly Caused by

- Spontaneous intracranial hemorrhage
- Head injury due to motor vehicle accidents, recreational, industrial accidents, gunshot assault, etc.
- Cerebral anoxia/ischemic injury (cardiac arrest due to asthma, asphyxiation, drug overdose, hanging, drowning, meningitis, carbon monoxide poisoning, or primary cardiac arrest)
- Primary cerebral tumour.

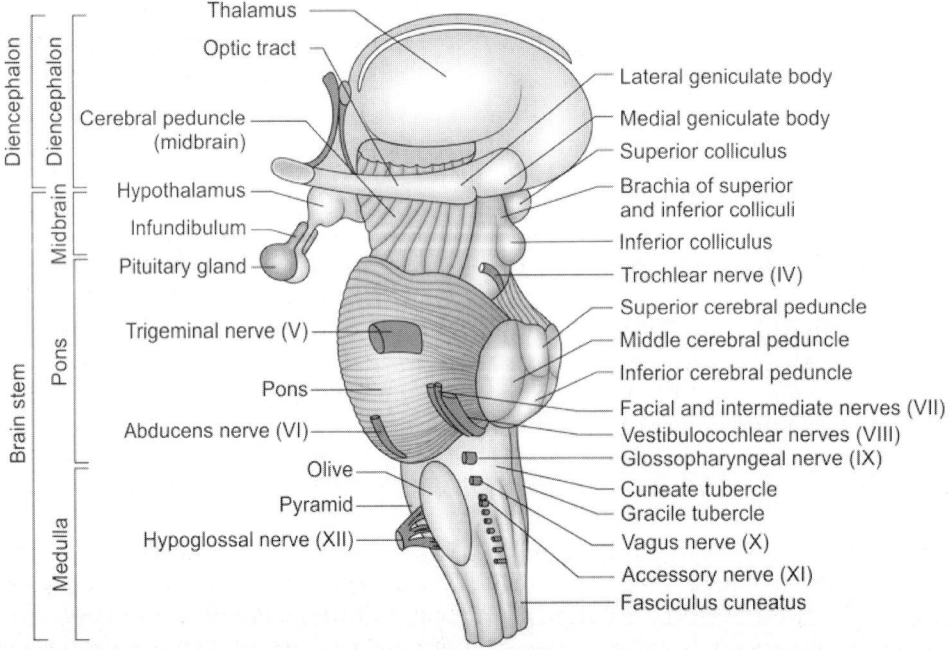

Fig. 2.1: Brain stem

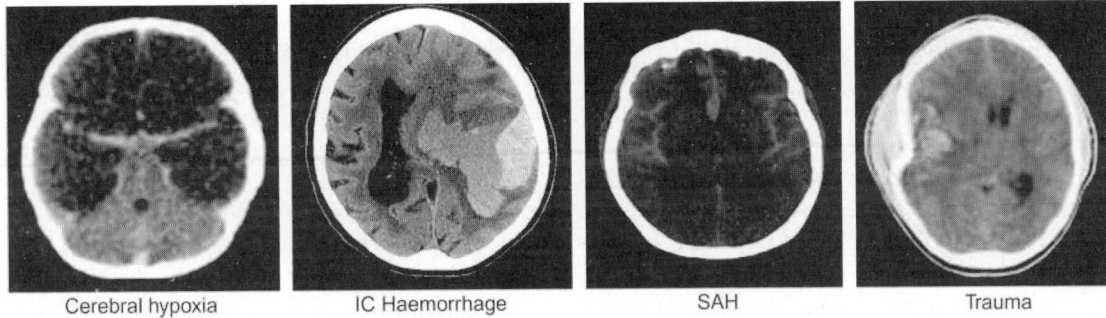

| Cerebral hypoxia | IC Haemorrhage | SAH | Trauma |

Fig. 2.2: Causes of brain death

Path Physiology of Brain Death

It is important to understand what happens in the brain that it progresses to brain death after a significant insult. There are a few concepts which one needs to understand

Brain is a Fixed Compartment Model

The skull which protects the brain acts like a fixed compartment, the volume inside it remaining constant. The contents in normal condition, the 3 main components are: Brain parenchyma ~80%, CSF ~10% and blood ~10%. If there is any change in the volume of

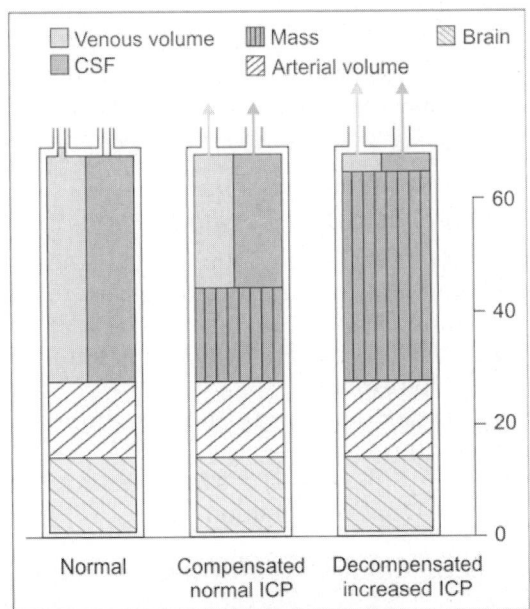

Fig. 2.3: Intracranial compensation for an expanding mass lesion

one of the 3 components, then it can only occur when one of the other components volume is reduced. The example been, if there is brain parenchyma swelling, then either CSF will be pushed out or blood flow to brain will be reduced to accommodate the increase in brain parenchyma volume due to swelling.

Cerebral Perfusion Pressure (CPP)

Often called CPP it is the pressure at which the brain is perfused with arterial blood. It is calculated as the difference between the mean arterial pressure (MAP) and the intracranial pressure (ICP). With the MAP being the mean blood pressure and ICP being the pressure within the skull which in normal circumstances is around the central venous pressure (CVP)

$$MAP - ICP = CPP$$

MAP is around 70 mm Hg, ICP is around 10 mm Hg

70 – 10 = 60 mm Hg is the normal CPP

These numbers are not absolute, hence a CPP between 50 mm Hg and 70 mm Hg is often considered to be within acceptable limits.

What happens during neuronal injury?

When there is a neuronal injury it results in neuronal swelling, which in turn causes a rise in intracranial pressure (ICP) and if this is not treated or does not respond to therapy, then it results in decrease in cerebral blood flow and decrease in cerebral perfusion pressure (CPP) which in turn causes further neuronal injury due to lack of oxygen, Thus a vicious cycle is established. Once the intracranial pressure

(ICP) rises above the mean arterial pressure (MAP), then there is no blood flow to the brain and all functions of brain stem are irreversibly ceased.

Simultaneously there is another process which happens as the neuronal swelling increases and that is called coning, as the swelling increases the only place for brain to expand is around the foramen magnum which is the opening at base of skull for spinal cord to continue. As this is the only opening the brain stem is pushed into the narrow opening which is conical in shape and hence called the coning of patient. Coning further hastens the lack of blood supply to brain stem and causes irreversible loss of brain stem functions.

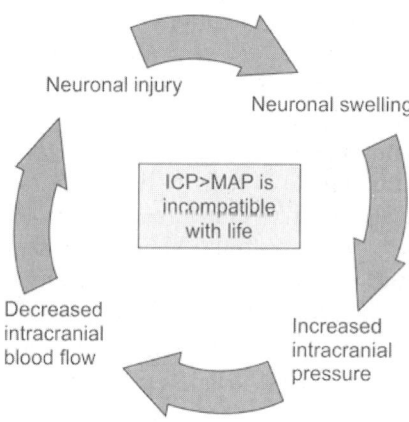

Fig. 2.4: Mechanism of cerebral death

Diagnosing Brain Death and Declaring Patient Dead

From the above discussion we understand that there should be a cause of irreversible coma, there are also certain preconditions which should be fulfilled before proceeding to diagnose brain death.

Preconditions

- Clear cause of irreversible coma (already discussed in detail above)
- Blood pressure above 90 mm Hg systolic and saturation >92%
- Temperature >35°C
- No toxins or poisons

- No sedatives or paralysing agents
- Metabolic and endocrine functions normal—especially no hypoglycaemia, hyponatremia, severe hypophosphatemia and severe hypothyroidism
- No brain stem infection like encephalitis or neurotoxins like snakebite, etc. (need to visit history again).

Once the preconditions are met then the brain death examination can be started once there are no observations noted of any breathing or brain stem activity by the bed side doctor and nurse for at least 4–6 hours.

As per our law

- 2 set of examinations are needed to diagnose brain death
- The time interval between the 2 examinations is 6 hours
- A neurologist, intensivist, neurosurgeon or an anesthesiologist usually are authorised to do the testing.
- One of the 2 tests should be done by a neurologist
- There are 2 other doctors who observe the test: Admitting physician and hospital administrator.
- All of the above doctors and administrators are usually pre-authorised from appropriate authority to conduct the examination.
- Time of death is the end of second apnoea test.

Practical Tips before Starting Testing

- Insist on core temperature measurement.
- Always look in history for drugs, overdose, sedation, etc.
- If available, use a peripheral nerve stimulator for TOF response.
- Have most recent values for sodium and potassium available.
- Insist on ABG at start of clinical testing with 100% O_2 pre-oxygenation.

1. Documentation of Irreversible Coma

- Absence of motor response to a standardized painful stimulus in cranial nerve distribution—acceptable is supraorbital pressure and trapezius muscle squeeze

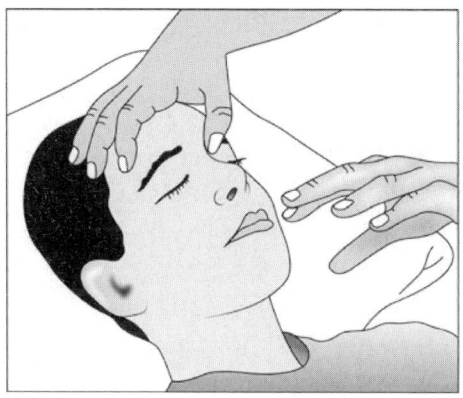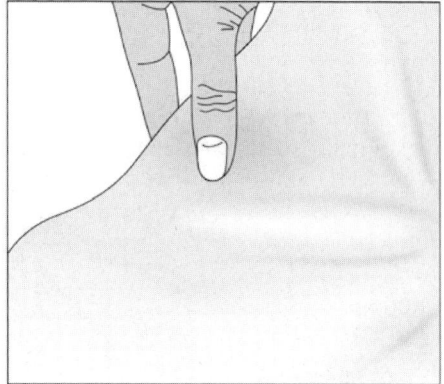

Fig. 2.5: Mechanism of cerebral death

• Beware of local spinal reflexes causing spontaneous or stimulus-related motor movements

2. Documentation of the Absence of Brain Stem Reflexes

• Brain stem reflexes are lost in a rostral-to-caudal direction
• Reflexes in medulla oblongata are the last to cease
• Tests documented are
  – Absent pupillary reflex
  – Absent oculocephalic movements (doll's eye reflex)
  – Absent oculovestibular reflex (cold calorie test)
  – Absent corneal reflex
  – Absent cough reflex

3. Documentation of Apnea (Apnea Test)

• Pre-oxygenation with 100% oxygen for at least 15 min.

• Give adequate volume and Vasopressors to keep MAP ~70 mm Hg
• CO_2 rises by around 3 mm HG/min of apnea, so be prepared to test at least for 8–10 min
  a. Preoxygenate patient with 100% oxygen for 15 minutes
  b. Obtain an ABG
  c. Disconnect patient from mechanical ventilation
  d. Continue to oxygenate through a catheter placed in the trachea—aim for saturation above 95%
  e. ABG is repeated within about 8–10 minutes
  f. Increase in $PaCO_2$ (above 60 mm Hg or 20 mm Hg from base line) and lack of respiration documented (use $EtCO_2$) if available

"Once the 2 specialists complete the test the time of death is confirmed as the end of second examination time".

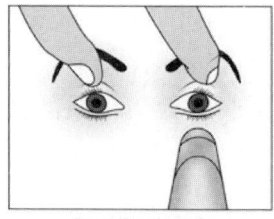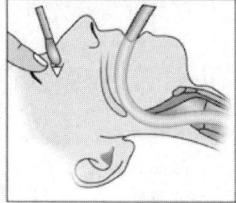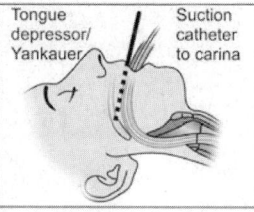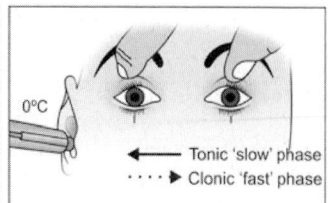

Tongue depressor/ Yankauer
Suction catheter to carina
0°C
Tonic 'slow' phase
Clonic 'fast' phase

Pupillary reflex   Corneal reflex   Cough and gag   Cold caloric test

Fig. 2.6

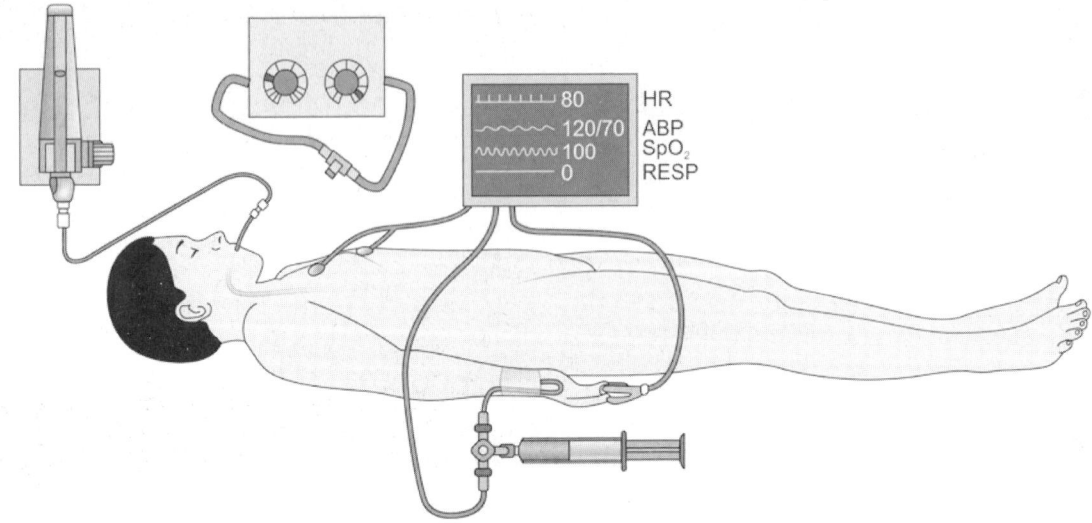

Fig. 2.7: Apnoea test

Ancillary or Radiographic Confirmation

Currently the THOA act is silent on the radiographic conformation of brain death. It is clear that the radiological test often referred as ancillary test is not a substitute to the clinical testing, however, in certain clinical scenarios or pediatric population, ancillary test would be important.

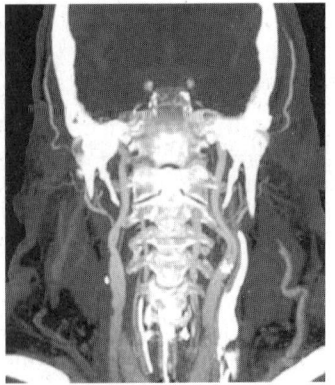

CT angiography

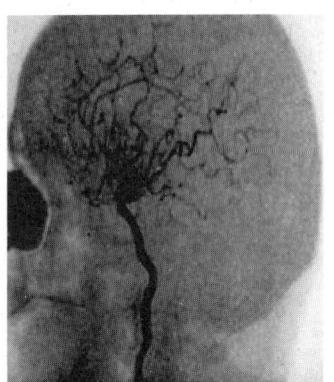

4-Vessel DSA

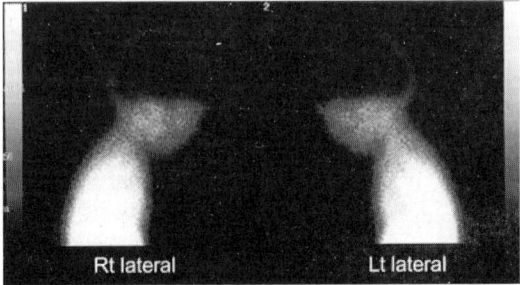

Rt lateral   Lt lateral

Radioactive perfusion scan

Fig. 2.8

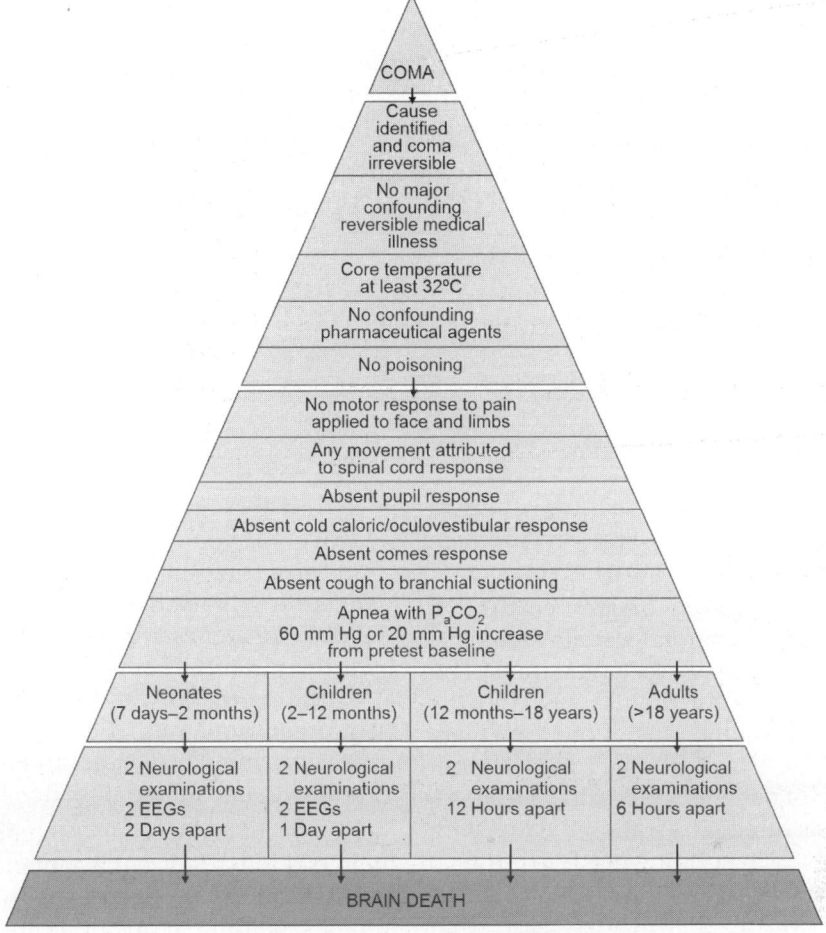

Fig. 2.9: Algorithm for BSD certification

Clinical Condition

- Testing is not complete or possible, i.e. facial fractures, swollen eyes, etc.
- Cervical spine fractures
- Apnea test becomes a challenge because of spinal fracture or severe hemodynamic compromise.

The acceptable ancillary test is

- CT angiography
- Four-vessel digital subtraction angiography
- Radioactive perfusion scan.

Though the law is silent these (ancillary) tests can be used along with the clinical testing whenever the complete clinical examination is not possible.

Further Reading

Donor management Guidelines are published by Indian Society of Critical Care Medicine (ISCCM), they can be downloaded from the following link

http://isccm.org/images/Management_of_Potential_Organ_Donor_final_IJCCM.pdf

Role of the Transplant Coordinator

Santosh Sarote

Transplant coordinators are involved in practically every aspect of organ procurement and transplantation. This may involve

- **Educating potential organ recipients:** Transplant coordinators educate recipients in how to best prepare for organ transplant and how to care for themselves after the transplant. The functions of the transplant coordinator are multiple. Right from admission of patients, contacting surgeons, anesthetists nurses, operation theatre staff, laboratory test everything needs to be taken care of. They help patients to get registered on organ waiting list. They ensure that patients have a support system of family, friends, and caregivers in place. They also play a role in the post-transplant recovery by arranging medicines, lab tests, visits to hospitals and by counselling regarding danger symptoms.
- **Counseling donor families:** Transplant coordinators also help the families of organ donor's deal with the death of their loved one and inform them of the organ donation process.

Once the donor patient has been declared brain dead and is no longer breathing on his or her own, the transplant coordinator approaches the donor's family about organ donation. If the family gives its consent, the coordinator then collects the necessary medical information and also calls the ZTCC, SOTTO, ROTTO or NOTTO office.

- **Record keeping:** Transplant coordinators are actively involved in evaluating, planning, and maintaining records and liasing with ZTCC regarding the patients on the waiting lists.
- **Public awareness:** Another significant aspect of the job of all transplant coordinators is educating the public about the importance of organ donation. They speak to hospital and nursing school staffs and to the general public to encourage donations.

Transplant coordinators can be found doing their jobs in various environments. The work schedule varies from office work, it includes visiting families, helping in doctor's clinic. They may have to accompany the patient in the hospital and work for long hours. They may be in an office completing paperwork, in a hospital visiting with patients, families, or other hospital staff, in a clinic or doctor's office seeing patients, or at a school or business meeting promoting donor awareness. Sometimes coordinators must accompany the organ to the transplant center, and some may be required to be on call and to work long, irregular hours. An important part of their job is helping individuals and families.

To be a successful transplant coordinator, one should have good organizational skills and be able to work quickly, accurately, and efficiently. You must be a detail-oriented person and have good record-keeping and reporting skills. The various skills required for this profession are compassion, good communication, record keeping and paper reportings.

Kidney

Anatomy, Physiology of Kidney and Diseases

Bhushan Patil

INTRODUCTION: ANATOMY OF KIDNEY

- The kidney is a reddish brown, bean-shaped organ with the dimensions 12 × 6 × 3 cm.
- Weight of kidney is approx. 125–150 gm
- Both kidneys are supplied by one renal artery which is branch of aorta, and drained by renal vein which merge with IVC
- Although they are similar in size and shape, the left kidney is slightly longer and more slender than the right kidney, and nearer to the midline.
- Each kidney has: Convex upper and lower ends, convex lateral border, convex medial border at both ends, but its middle shows a vertical slit called the hilum.
- The hilum transmits from anterior to posterior, the renal vein, renal artery and the ureter. Lymph vessels and sympathetic fibers also pass through the hilum.

   Internally the hilum extends into a large cavity called the renal sinus.

   Each kidney consists of an outer renal cortex and an inner renal medulla.

- The renal cortex is a continuous band of pale tissue that completely surrounds the renal medulla.
- Extensions of the renal cortex, the renal columns project into the inner aspect of the kidney, dividing the renal medulla into discontinuous aggregations of triangular-shaped tissue, the renal pyramids (Fig. 1.1).

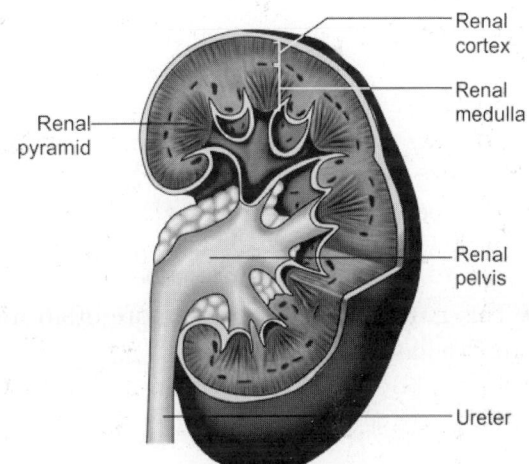

Fig. 1.1: Anatomy of the kidney

- The renal artery arises from the aorta at the level of the second lumbar vertebra. *So, for this reason the left kidney is the preferred side for live donor nephrectomy. The site of entry of left renal vein into IVC is above the right renal vein. The right renal vein is behind the 2nd part of the duodenum and sometimes behind the lateral part of the head of the pancreas.*
- The structural and functional units of the kidneys are nephrons responsible for forming urine. Main structures of the nephrons (Fig. 1.2).
   - Glomerulus
   - Renal tubule
- Most people are born with 2 kidneys. But sometimes the kidneys form fused together.

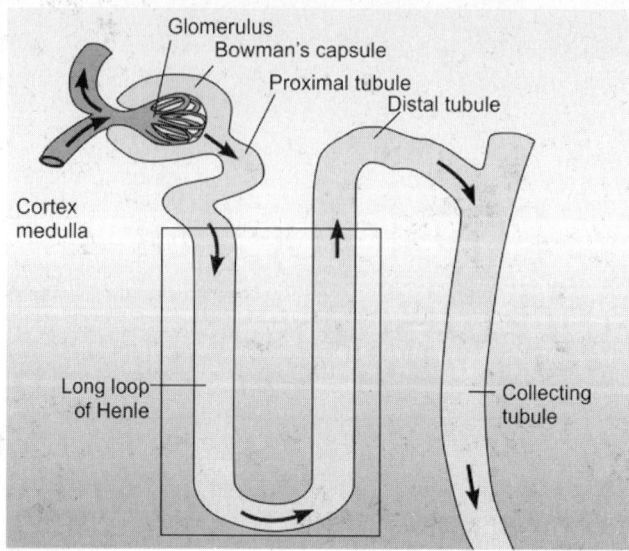

Fig. 1.2: Horseshoe kidney

It occurs during fetal development as the kidneys move into their normal position.

- They become attached ("fuse") together at the lower end or base. By fusing, they form into a U-shape, like a horseshoe.
- This is thought to happen more often in males than in females.
- Horseshoe kidney occurs in about 1 in 500 children (Fig. 1.3).

Anatomy of Ureter

These are slender tubes attaching the kidney to the bladder

- Continuous with the renal pelvis
- Enter the posterior aspect of the bladder

Anatomy of Urinary Bladder

- It is smooth, collapsible, muscular sac
- It temporarily stores urine.

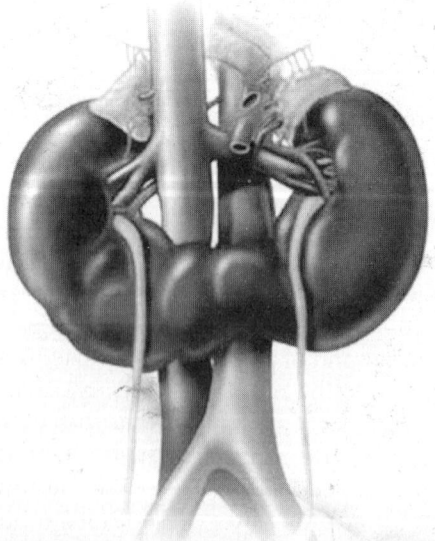

Fig. 1.3: Pictorial depiction of glomerulus and collecting system of kidney

Functions of the Urinary System (Fig. 1.4)

- Regulating blood volume and pressure
- Regulating plasma concentrations of sodium, potassium, chloride and other ions
- Stabilising blood pH
- Conserving nutrients
- Detoxifying poisons (with the liver)
- Some reabsorption is passive, most is active, it requires energy.
- Most reabsorption occurs in the proximal convoluted tubule
- Nitrogenous waste products like urea, uric acid, creatinine

Secretion: Some materials move from the peritubular capillaries into the renal tubules, e.g. hydrogen, potassium ions and creatinine.

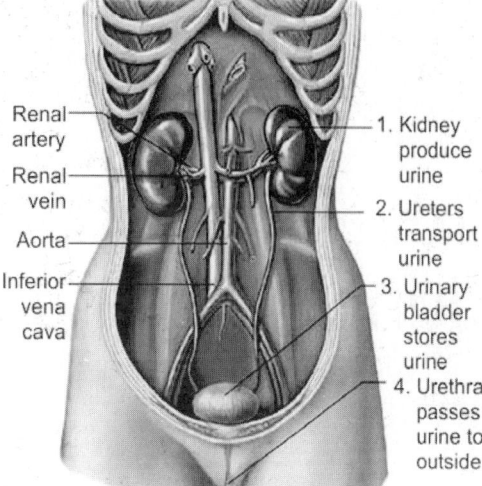

Renal artery

Renal vein

Aorta

Inferior vena cava

1. Kidney produce urine
2. Ureters transport urine
3. Urinary bladder stores urine
4. Urethra passes urine to outside

Fig. 1.4: The urinary system

Prevention of Kidney Disease

Tukaram Jamale

Who is at Risk of Chronic Kidney Disease?

About 17% of Indian adults have chronic kidney disease. Who is at risk of kidney disease? The major risk factors contributing are: Diabetes, high BP and family history of renal failure. In addition, history of kidney stones, regular use of certain pain killer medications, past history of kidney disease as a child also increases your risk.

What are the Symptoms Associated with Kidney Disease?

It is a common misconception that patients with kidney disease will always have decrease in urine production, or swelling on their feet. Kidney disease often has no symptoms, and it can go undetected until very advanced stage. But a simple urine test can tell you if you have kidney disease. Remember, it is important to get tests done, because early detection and treatment can slow or prevent the pro-gression of kidney disease. This doesn't mean that each one of us should rush to get tested.

Who Should Get Regular Testing?

Testing is needed for those with increased risk of kidney disease like: Diabetes, high blood pressure, kidney stones, previous or childhood history of kidney disease, family history of kidney disease. Diagnosing kidney disease needs simple laboratory tests that are widely available like urine examination serum creatinine. You will be advised about further testing by your kidney doctor.

How can Kidney Failure be Prevented?

Diabetes and high blood pressure are leading causes of kidney failure worldwide and strict control of both of these is the most important step to prevent kidney failure. Both of these conditions are generally silent, i.e. will not produce symptoms until very high. Only way to ensure their appropriate control is to periodically check it and be in follow-up of your physician who will modify treatment if needed. Same holds true about kidney stones, which is one of the leading causes of kidney failure. Everyone with history of kidney stones, should get their blood and urine tests regularly in addition to annual ultrasonography. Early detection and appropriate treatment at this stage is important to prevent kidney failure.

Chronic kidney disease (CKD) range from very mild damage to kidney (stage 1) to dialysis requiring kidney failure (stage 5). If you get detected in earlier stages, appropriate treatment can be started to slow or prevent the progression of the disease to kidney failure stage. Many patients with CKD, detected and treated early, may never need dialysis or kidney transplant in their life and can be managed with appropriate medications. Having known that one has got CKD, many patients resort to alternative therapies which are not only unproven but also can be dangerous as some of them can accelerate the disease progression. Also, crucial time in the early stages of CKD is lost, when treatment to retard the progression of the disease is most effective.

Pre-transplant Medical Work up of Kidney Recipient

NK Hase

INTRODUCTION

Renal transplant is the preferred treatment for end stage renal disease. A successful renal transplant improves the quality of life and reduces the mortality risk for most patients, when compared with maintenance dialysis. There is however, a shortage of donated organs and a growing waiting list for transplantation. It is important to evaluate potential renal transplant recipient carefully to detect and treat co-existing illness which may affect survival after transplantation.

1. Who should be Evaluated for Placing on Waiting List for Transplantation?

Patients who have severe chronic renal failure with GFR less than 10 ml/min or patients who are on haemodialysis or peritoneal dialysis and have expressed an interest in undergoing renal transplant, are jointly evaluated by nephrologists and the transplant surgeon at outpatient clinic. The transplant coordinator plays a pivotal role in the whole process of evaluation.

2. What are the Aims of Evaluation?

a. To rule out underlying diseases that may be exacerbated by surgery or immuno-suppressive drugs.
b. To rule out original disease that may recur in the transplanted kidney.
c. Educate and evaluate patients about socio-economic and psychologic aspects.

d. To rule out acute active infections and contraindication for transplantation.

The **renal transplant evaluation** should begin with a brief history and physical examination, so that obvious contraindication to transplantation can be detected before expensive and invasive tests are obtained.

History and physical examination for

- Determining the underlying cause of renal failure
- Complications of renal failure that are present.
- Detection of co-morbid factors like anaemia, hypertension diabetes, cardiovascular, respiratory, gastrointestinal diseases, renal bone disease and peripheral neuropathy.
- History of previous urinary tract infections, tuberculosis, hepatitis, dental, skin infection and infection at any other site.
- History of stone disease, operation done, etiology of stone disease.
- Family history—renal diseases, diabetes and hypertension.

Current Clinical Data and Treatment

Type of dialysis, duration, frequency of dialysis, dialysis related complications, state of vascular access, hepatitis vaccination, pneumococcal and influenza, varicella vaccination, control of BP, interdialysis weight gain, dry weight, number of blood transfusion received, diet, drug and native kidney urine output.

Initial Laboratory Evaluation

- **Haematological evaluation:** Complete blood count Hb, PCV, WBC, DC blood group, BT, CT, PTT, PT, fibrinogen.
- **Renal:** Urine—routine and culture and colony count. 24 hours urinary proteins, urinary protein/creatinine ratio, BUN, serum creatinine, serum uric acid, serum Na, K, Cl, HCO_3, serum Ca, P, O_4, alkaline phosphatase, PTH and vitamin D_3.
- **Liver function tests:** Direct, indirect and total serum bilirubin, ALT, AST and serum proteins
- **Metabolic and endocrine:** Blood glucose fasting and PP, serum cholesterol, TG (lipid profile)
- **Serological and immunological:** HBsAg, HCV antibodies, HCV-RNA titres, HIV antibodies, cytomegalovirus, herpes simplex, EBV and varicella antibody testing, VDRL, RA, HLA typing and panel reactive antibody to detect for previous sensitization.
- Serum PSA if age > 50 years.
- **Radiological:** X-ray chest PA, plain KUB, USG abdomen and pelvis, colour Doppler for aortic, renal, iliac, femoral and carotid vessels.
- **Cardiac evaluation:** ECG, 2D ECHO, coronary angiography as indicated, stress test
- **Assessment of lower urinary tract:** Urine flowmetry, postvoid residue, voiding—cystourethrogram and cystoscopy in selected cases.
- **Dental skin and ENT evaluation:** To r/o mainly septic foci.
- **Psychiatric evaluation:** Personality trend and to rule out non-compliance and substance abuse.
- **In women gynaecological check includes:** Pap smear, breast examination and mammography if age more than 40 years
- **Miscellaneous:** Gastroscopy, colonoscopy in selected cases where history of peptic ulcer and stool occult blood is positive. Social worker evaluation about economic, social and financial states.

Once the above information is gathered and there are no contraindications to transplant, a meeting is set up with the patient and his or her family, the transplant surgeon, the transplant nephrologists and anesthesiologists. The patient is placed on waiting list of the hospital and the form duly endorsed by head of the institution is sent to ROTTO to add to city waiting list.

Maintenance of Current Register of Prospective Kidney Recipients

Sr. No.

Name

Age

Sex

Address

Telephone No: Residence .... Office........

Mobile..................... Pager..........................

Information needed to keep the register up to date

3 monthly Evaluation   Clinical evaluation

Monthly Evaluation   Hemoglobin

    Total and differential count

    ESR

    Urine routine and microscopy, urine culture

    Liver function test

    Serum calcium, phosphorus and uric acid

    Blood sugars

    HIV

    HbsAg, HBsAb

Certification of a Prospective Recipient

This is to certify that Mr/Mrs .... is suffering from chronic renal failure, end stage renal disease and is on maintenance dialysis at hospital. He/she does not have a prospective live related kidney donor and is therefore registered for a deceased kidney donor transplant, the procedure involved, the cost of undergoing the deceased donor transplant and maintenance immuno-suppression have all been explained to her/him. He/she is obliged to report to this hospital immediately on being informed of the availability of a suitable deceased donor. It is mandatory for her to keep this hospital informed in the event of her/him leaving the city for any duration of time.

Information to be Maintained

Residential address and telephone number of recipient/guardian

Office address and telephone number of recipient

Mobile/Pager number of recipient/guardian

Change in address/Telephone/Mobile no.

Counselling of recipients on

1. Emergency nature of surgery
2. After being called for transplant and reaching the centre also probable chance of disappointment due to medical unfitness.
3. Rate of complications.
4. Possibility of DGF along with post-op dialysis.
5. Immunosuppression drugs.
6. Lifelong drugs and precautions.
7. Financial arrangements.

Financial Arrangements

Depending upon the hospital, cost may vary which the patient must be aware of and be ready. In case of any complication cost too will spiral up.

Management Protocol on Availability of a Prospective Deceased Donor

Contact patient

Cross check blood group

Admit in Nephrology ward

Send routine investigations—CBC, BUN, creatinine, LFT, Ca, PO_4, UA, blood glucose—random, urine routine, urine culture, blood group, X-ray and ECG, BT, PT, PTTK, platelet count.

Collect blood of donor for HLA and lymphocyte cross match.

Start dialysis: New dialyser fluid, tubing, and fistula puncture needles if needed.

4 hours dialysis

Post dialysis BUN, creatinine CBC, electrolytes

Isolation of patient

Immunosuppression

As per protocol of unit

Antibiotics as per protocol

Give drug prescription

Blood arrangement 3 pints

To make theatre arrangements cleaning and fumigation of post-operative recovery room.

Call to anesthetist and physician.

Consent in special form

After the dialysis if lymphocyte cross match is negative, then preoperative orders are given as per protocol of unit

NBM to be continued.

Shave from nipple to knee

Simple enema

Clean hot water bath with hair shampooing

Immunosuppression as per protocol

Fresh electrolyte report

Shift patient to theatre.

Post-renal Transplant Medications and Precautions

MM Bahadur

Renal transplant is an operation where a genetically different kidney (allograft) is placed within a recipient to replace the function of the diseased one. Since even the best matched allograft is not an exact genetic match to the recipient it is recognized as 'foreign' by the body of the recipient and a process of rejection starts immediately and continues lifelong. This process needs to be suppressed by a combination of anti-rejection drugs which makes the recipient to accept the allograft but it comes with a necessary evil-predisposition to infections by reducing the immunity of the individual significantly.

Unlike liver, which is relatively a more tolerant organ requiring less immunosuppression, kidney does not achieve tolerance even years and decades after transplantation. Hence significant lifelong immunosuppression is a must. Even decades later any noncompliance of anti-rejection medications can lead to rejection of the transplanted kidney. This truth needs to be emphasized repeatedly to the transplant recipient, specially to the young, teenage patients who are most likely to be non-compliant.

Kidney allograft recipient requires triple drug immunosuppression. The drug regimen usually consists of at least one drug from each group given below:

- Steroid (Prednisolone, Deflazocort).
- CNI inhibitor—Calcineurin inhibitor—Tacrolimus, Cyclosporin
- Antimetabolite—Mycophenolate Moefitil, Azathioprine
- Sometimes the CNI inhibitor is replaced by mTOR inhibitor such as, Sirolimus or Everolimus.

In certain transplant centers induction immunosuppression is used in addition to the drugs in the form of injectable ATG or injectable Basiliximab pre-transplant in all cases. At other centers it is used selectively for high risk cases like sensitized individuals, poor genetic match and spousal transplants.

In the first few months prophylaxis has to be given for some infections which reside in the body such as cytomegalovirus (CMV), *Pneumocystis carinii* pneumonia (PCP), etc. but manifest as disease only when high dose immunosuppression is given in the early days post-transplant. These include acyclovir and septran. This is specially so if induction has been used in the form of injectable ATG or injectable Basiliximab pre-transplant.

Each group of drugs act at different sites of the rejection cascade and hence act synergistically to each other enhancing the blockade of the rejection cycle.

Besides the anti-rejection medicines, they generally require some medicines for blood pressure control and if they are diabetic either insulin injections or oral anti-diabetic medications or both.

Some calcium and vitamin preparations are also required for their well-being.

Even though transplant patients lead a normal healthy life they need to keep a few things in mind. It would make sense to reinforce the precautions listed below:

1. Anti-rejection medicines are for lifetime. Even a single dose cannot be missed. In case of accidental dose lapse or vomiting, unable to take medicines for whatever reason contact your nephrologist.

2. Do not change the dose, frequency and brand of medications or add and subtract medicines without consulting your doctor, for reduced or increased drug bio-availability of drugs can alter graft functions permanently.

3. Regular periodic lab checks, renal bio-chemistry and follow-up with the doctor is mandatory even if one is feeling fine and even if the transplant is several decades old or longer.

4. Drug levels when ordered by the doctor to adjust drug doses are trough levels (Tacrolimus level or cyclosporine or sirolimus levels), i.e. when blood is to be drawn before the next dose of that medicines.

5. Strict hygienic practices to be followed lifelong.

6. Boiled cooled water and home cooked food is preferred otherwise food consumed need to be hygienically prepared, stored and served because acute gut infections are the commonest infections in India in the post-transplant period. Any infection is potentially harmful to the graft and serious infections can lead to either graft loss or death.

7. Pre-transplant vaccinations and post-transplant boosters where indicated should be taken. As a rule, only dead or subunit vaccines (not live attenuated ones) are permissible in the post-transplant period.

8. Keep away from potentially infected people, e.g. those having severe cold, don't be shy to use a mask in crowded places and take precautions to prevent infection, for a simple infection in a immunocompetent individual can be life-threatening in a transplant individual. Treat all infections, fevers, loose motions, cough as serious and take doctors' advice.

9. Do not take NSAID's pain killers, anti-biotics, alternative medications on your own.

With modern medicines and due care by the patient, one can expect him to live a long fruitful life.

Swap Renal Transplantation in Mumbai

Ganesh Sanap, Deepa Usulumarty, Viswanath Billa

A Swap transplant, or Paired exchange transplant, involves an exchange of organs between two families, who cannot donate the organ to their own family member because of blood group mismatch or tissue incompatibilities. This in simplistic terms is a 'paired exchange'. By doing a swap, two patients with kidney failure, who, under normal circumstances cannot undergo a transplant because of blood group mismatch within that family, can now go ahead with kidney transplantation. Felix Rapaport first suggested the concept of a swap transplant in 1986. The first paired transplants were conducted in South Korea in 1991. Switzerland and USA performed their first paired kidney exchange (PKE) in 1999 and 2000, respectively. Since then, it has gained popularity across the globe.

Types of Swaps

1. 2-way exchange (Binary swap)
2. 3-way exchange
3. List exchange
4. Domino paired donation
5. NEAD model

Binary Swap Kidney Transplant *(Fig. 5.1)*

The most basic exchange between incompatible pairs is through a two-way exchange, where two incompatible pairs with reciprocal incompatibilities are paired up and kidneys are swapped. In this model, the donor from the first pair donates to the recipient of the

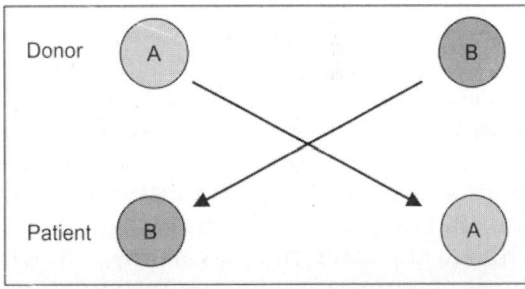

Fig. 5.1: Binary swap kidney transplant

second pair and the donor from the second pair donates to their recipient of the first pair. Thus, both recipients benefit from a live donation indirectly through their willing but incompatible donor.

Three-way Exchanges

Three-way exchanges are built upon the foundation of two-way exchanges by including an additional incompatible pair. This approach not only increases the number of transplants possible but also facilitates better outcomes for hard-to-match pairs by not requiring reciprocal matching. For example, in a two-way exchange, an O recipient has difficulty not just in finding a compatible donor but in also finding a compatible donor whose incompatible recipient can receive a kidney from the O recipient's incompatible donor. A three-way exchange eases this burden by including another incompatible pair that overcomes this need for reciprocity.

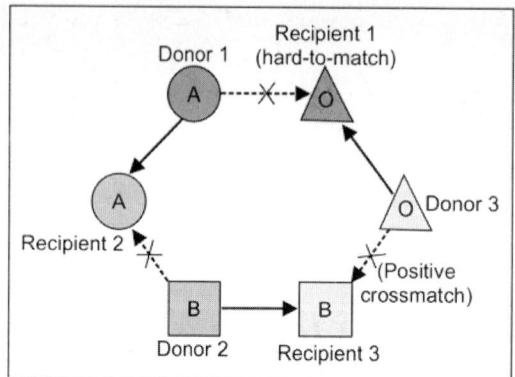

Fig. 5.2: Three-way exchange

List Exchange

In a list exchange an incompatible living donor donates to a candidate waiting for a deceased donor kidney, and in exchange, the recipient from the incompatible pair acquires priority on the wait-list for a future deceased donor organ. This model is successful in its ability to facilitate an additional transplant through the generosity of the willing donor, while at the same time awarding a much shorter waiting time for the incompatible recipient. However, many fear list exchanges promote an unacceptable disadvantage to blood type O candidates on the wait-list since the most common list exchange would involve non-blood type O donor kidneys being exchanged for blood type O deceased donor kidneys.

Domino Paired Donation

A donor who is incompatible with his recipient gives to the recipient of another incompatible

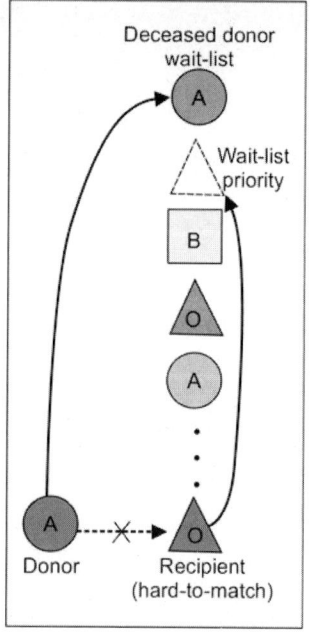

Fig. 5.3: List exchange

pair. In return, the donor of that incompatible pair extends the chain by donating to another recipient of an incompatible pair. This can theoretically go on to include several such mutually incompatible pairs. The last donor donates to the first recipient of the chain and the loop ends. Thus, narrow mutual incompatibilities can be converted into broad systematic compatibilities for the benefit of all.

Non-Simultaneous Extended Altruistic Donor (NEAD) Model

A NEAD chain is similar to a Domino chain with some significant differences. In this an

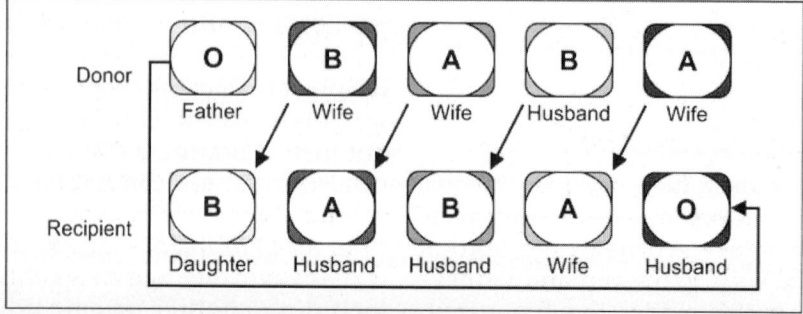

Fig. 5.4: Domino paired donation

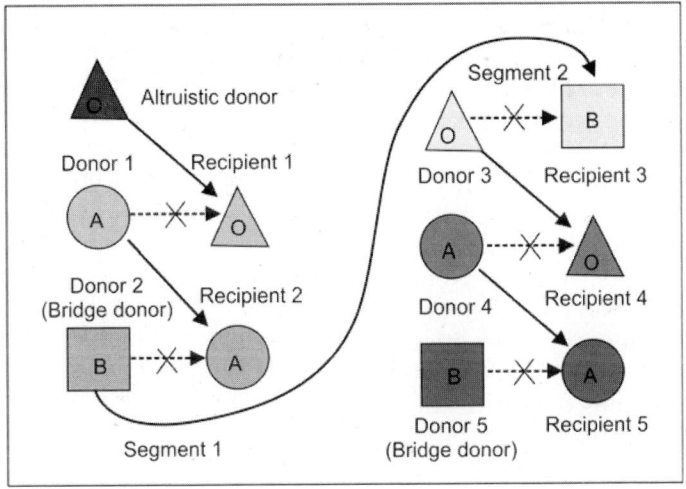

Fig. 5.5: NEAD chain

altruistic donor initiates the chain. The subsequent transplants are not performed simultaneously. Being non-simultaneous, this chain length can become very large since there are no limitations imposed by the lack of being simultaneous. There is however a risk of donor back tracking on his commitment and hence these transplants need to be evaluated very carefully.

Situations where Swaps Transplants can be Considered

- Patients with kidney failure who have a blood group incompatible donor
- Patients with kidney failure who have a blood group compatible donor, but their lymphocyte crossmatch is positive.
- Patients with kidney failure who have a suitable donor within the family, but such a donor has tested positive for Hepatitis B or C. Such patients may enter the swap registry to find a potential recipient who is also seropositive for the similar virus.
- Patients who have elderly donors with a compatible group register to get a better age-matched donor. For example—Mr. "X" a dialysis patient with blood group B is compatible with his father with blood group O. He preferentially registers for a swap transplant to get a better age matched donor

younger than his father. Such a situation is a win-win for patient X, as well as those patients with 'difficult to match' blood group O recipients.

Experience of Paired Kidney Transplants in Mumbai

There are different NGOs in Mumbai that keep a record of incompatible donor recipient pairs in their database. Notable among these are:

1. Apex swap transplant registry
2. Narmada kidney foundation

The Apex Swap Transplant Registry (ASTRA)—an initiative of Apex Kidney Foundation started its swap transplant registry. Since inception more than 350 donor-recipient pairs have been registered for a swap transplant. From this database, 53 paired kidney transplants have been completed successfully. ASTRA has developed a mathematical model in collaboration with IIT Mumbai and leverages this algorithm to find a solution for the problem of organ shortage. The country's first transplant in a complex domino loop of 5 donor-recipient pairs was performed in 2013 followed by a 6 pair domino kidney swap transplantation which is the longest such chain in Asia to date. This was performed out of the ASTRA database.

Paired Kidney Exchange vs ABOi Transplants

There is a huge demand and supply mismatch for living-related donors. Many of the living related donors who get rejected is because of ABO incompatibility (ABOi) or a positive crossmatch between the donor and recipient. It has been shown that such incompatibilities can account for the rejection of up to 35% of otherwise suitable donors. To circumvent this problem, various alternatives have been devised such as ABOi transplants and desensitization protocols for patients with a positive cross-match. Patients undergoing desensitization or ABOi transplants require plasmapheresis sessions as well as a considerably higher requirement of immunosuppression including rituximab, thymoglobulin, over and above the regular maintenance immunosuppression. Finally, these options are significantly more expensive compared to conventional transplants. While ABO incompatible transplants are possible nowadays with advances in immunosuppression, there still exist a higher chance of infections and rejections with such transplants, aside from the significantly higher cost. Therefore, a paired kidney exchange (PKE) program is definitely a simpler alternative for such patients. This is also reflected in the latest amendment of Transplantation of Human Organs (THO) Act 2011. There is an urgent need for a national level PKE program with a national PKE registry to promote better matching and increase number of patients benefiting from it.

Need for a Central Registry

India has approximately 180–200 kidney transplant centers and one-third of these are in the major metropolitan cities, mostly in the private sector. In the government-run tertiary care hospitals, maintenance dialysis, transplantation, and follow-up are conducted free of cost for the underprivileged section of the community. In the private system, there are two arrangements: One where transplantation is performed for a cost, which is nonprofit-oriented, and other where it is performed in corporate hospitals where the cost of transplantation and follow-up is high

for the average Indian patient. In India, most of the KT relies on live donor transplantation; however, many states have established a strong cadaveric transplantation program, one such example is Tamil Nadu Cadaver Transplant Programme, which is the most efficient and effective. Many other nongovernment organizations (NGOs) have established organ sharing networks, which promote the deceased donation program. The Foundation for Organ Transplantation and Education (Bangalore), Multi Organ Harvesting Aid Network, Narmada Kidney Foundation, Zonal Transplant Coordination Committee (Mumbai), Organ Retrieval Banking Organization (Delhi), and Delhi Organ Procurement Network and Transplant Education are some of the active groups.

The Prerequisites for a Swap Registry

A swap transplant registry needs to have a basic framework for data collection as well as storage. Additionally, it needs to address the needs of the society by certain foundational principles which need to be built into the exchange algorithm.

An allocation system that focuses on improving outcomes (graft survival, post-transplant performance) is considered a utility based system, and a system that prioritizes equal access regardless of need is an equity-based system. Since these are polar end approaches for allocation of any scarce resource, almost all references agree that good balance must be achieved in them. Such a balance must be achieved with a broader discussion with all stakeholders to get their inputs on the optimal weightage for the specific variables being considered.

Due prioritization and scoring is given to donor-recipient pairs based on recipient waiting period on dialysis, history of multiple access failure, previous failed transplant, recipient sensitization, HLA match with prospective pairs and period from registration in the swap registry. The matching algorithm should also include the native incompatible donors GFR and donor-recipient age difference to ensure that the matching is fair. The parameter of matching the location of the patient in relation to the donor includes taking care of logistics issues (particularly in India) associated with kidney transplants. Due to poor health, bad transportation and financial difficulties, many patients are unwilling to travel which makes any swap opportunity outside their region challenging.

Conclusion

Paired kidney donation is rapidly expanding for facilitating living donor renal transplantation for patients who are incompatible with their healthy, willing donors, increase in living donation rates. An annual exponential increase in percentages of swap transplants may be possible if donor-exchange programs were available nationwide. Comparatively short waiting time in KPD will save the cost of maintenance dialysis and associated morbidity and mortality. The constraints in operating an effective maintenance dialysis program leave renal transplants the only viable option for patients with ESRD in developing countries like India. In view of the cost and concerns regarding higher risks of infection and outcome of ABO incompatible renal transplant in a resource limited, developing country like ours, PKE is a more viable legal option. PKE should increase donor pool, thus preventing commercial transplantation. An active initiative by the government in setting up a national level registry to facilitate paired donations will go a long way. Swap kidney transplants are a viable, feasible and simple solution to ameliorate the shortage of organs in this country.

Liver, Pancreas and Bowel

Anatomy, Physiology of Liver and Multi-organ Retrieval

Fysal Kollanta Valappil

INTRODUCTION

The liver is the largest organ in the body weighing 1.2 to 1.6 kg, largely occupying the right upper quadrant. Liver is central to many main metabolic pathways and is essential for human survival. In an hepatic state human can survive only up to 48 hours. The liver possesses the unique ability to regenerate within a brief period.

ANATOMY OF THE LIVER

Embryologically, the liver is a foregut structure. It is composed of right and left lobe which is fixed in the right upper quadrant of the abdomen by peritoneal reflections called ligaments. The diaphragmatic peritoneal duplications are coronary ligaments whose lateral margins on either side are left and right triangular ligaments. Falciform ligament emerges from the centre of coronary ligament which runs to umbilicus. Functional anatomy of liver is composed of eight segments each supplied by single portal triad (portal vein, hepatic artery, bile duct). Cantlie's line which contains middle hepatic vein which runs from gallbladder fossa to the left of vena cava and divides the liver into right and left hemi livers.

The right liver is divided into anterior sector (5 and 8 segment) and posterior sector (6 and 7 segment). Left liver divided into left anterior sector (3 and 4 segment) and left posterior sector (segment 2). The caudate lobe is the dorsal portion of the liver. Blood supply of the liver being derived 80% from the portal vein and 20% from the hepatic artery. Portal vein divided into main right and left branch at the hilum of the liver. Hepatic artery which arises from the coeliac trunk gives right and left hepatic artery. The three major hepatic veins (the right, left and middle) drain directly into the inferior vena cava (IVC). The left hepatic vein usually joins middle hepatic vein intrahepatically and entering into the IVC. The right and left hepatic duct from the respective side of the liver joins to form the common hepatic duct.

Physiology of Liver

The functional unit of the liver is called an acinus or liver lobule. Liver is the centre of metabolic homeostasis and regulate energy metabolism. Liver synthesizes substantial number of proteins, enzymes, and vitamins, detoxifies and eliminates many exogenous and endogenous substances. Bile production (approximately 1500 ml) and secretion is one of the major functions of the liver. Bile helps to dispose the substance secreted into the bile and provides enteric bile salt to aid in the digestion of fats. Enterohepatic circulation of bile constitutes the major mechanism for eliminating excess cholesterol. Bile salts play critical role in the absorption of dietary fats and fat-soluble vitamins. Liver can store glucose in the form of glycogen and can give glucose for systemic circulation. Fatty acids are synthesised in the liver during the state of glucose excess, when the liver's ability to store glycogen been exceeded. During lipolysis free fatty acids are transported to liver where they are metabolised. Liver is needed for the synthesising most of the coagulation factors, for maintaining core body temperature, pH balance, correction of lactic acidosis, synthesis of urea.

Summary

A precise knowledge of the anatomy of the liver is an absolute prerequisite to perform successful surgery on the liver. The unique ability of liver to regenerate and its various synthetic and detoxifying functions reveals its importance.

MULTI-ORGAN PROCUREMENT FROM DECEASED DONOR

Advancement to modern day status of deceased donor organ procurement was aided in large part by work done in organ preservation and the acceptance of donation after brain death. Increased demand for donor organs has resulted in a concomitant increase in the use of marginal donors. Organ can be harvested from either from brainstem dead, heart beating donors/ donation after brain death (DBD) or from non-heart beating donors/donation after cardiac death (DCD). The organ procurement may be standard, rapid or super rapid depending on stable or urgent clinical circumstances or in arrested/non-heart beating donors.

Donor coordinator play a key role in

- Identification and selection of the potential donor
- Review and procurement of the appropriate and prescribed medical, legal and social consent from donor family
- Support and advice surrounding donor care in intensive care unit (ICU)
- Evaluation of the potential risk for the recipient
- Arrangement of the practical procedures involving the anaesthetist, the organ retrieval operation and sometimes

pathologist, bacteriologist and radiologist support as well as the donor ICU

- Coordination of land/air transportation for the procurement team
- Support of the medical and nursing staff in the operating theatre throughout the process of procurement up to, and including, the packaging and labelling of specimens
- Delivery of blood and tissue specimens to laboratories after the removal of the organs
- Distribution of donated organs to the appropriate transplant acceptor centres
- Logistics concerning the return (repatriation) of the retrieval team
- Advice and support to families before and after donation
- Feedback to the family, donor hospital staff and to the organ retrieval team(s)

All donors are tested for HIV I and II Ab, CMV-Ab, HbsAg, Toxoplasma-Ab, HBc-Ab, VDRL, antiHCV-Ab. The lead surgeon of the retrieval team and the coordinator are responsible for performing a risk assessment of the donor to determine any factor that might contribute to an increased risk of transfer of infection or malignancy to the recipient.

Before starting the retrieval, the team leader must check the following:
a. Brain death criteria are satisfied and recorded correctly
b. Cause of death
c. Consent for organ donation signed by the next of kin and coroner/police consent.
d. Relevant history and medication; history of jaundice, malignancy, diabetes hypertension, risk factors for transmission of malignancy, risk factors for transmission of viral and other infections, episode of cardio-respiratory arrest or instability, sepsis, hypoxia, hypotension, inotrope support, urine output (last hour and past 24 hours), blood group, virology, liver and renal function tests

Retrieval team

1. **Lead surgeon:** Liver team
2. **Assistant surgeon:** Renal team
3. **Additional cardiac team:** Two surgeons and operating room technician

4. Anaesthetist
5. Scrub nurse
6. Perfusionist
7. Coordinator

The perfusionist ensures that perfusion and other fluids are kept chilled in an ice box. These include 12 litres of HTK chilled, 2 litres of normal saline chilled and 4 litres of frozen normal saline. (Alternatively, centres using University of Wisconsin solution (UW) need to carry 6 litres of UW). The ice box should contain flaked ice to the brim and pressure infusion bags. The perfusionist also helps set up lines with the aortic line pressure infusion bag at 100 mm Hg and the portal line without pressure, changes the fluids as they finish and assist the scrub nurse on the back table with the back-table perfusion and in packing the organs.

The Donor Operation

1. Discuss plans for the operation with the anaesthetist and renal teams regarding incision and sternotomy, heparinization, aortic clamping, IVC clamping, bleed out
2. The order of organ retrieval is as follows— first heart/lung then liver, pancreas/ intestine, kidneys and corneas
3. Request the anaesthetist
   a. *To take a blood sample*: 2 × 20 ml = 40 ml for all tests. (Ensure 2 ml reaches blood bank for irregular antibody test).
   b. Administer intravenous antibiotic
   c. Muscle relaxant
   d. *Prepare for heparinization*: 300 units/kg
4. *Position patient*: Supine with arms by the side
5. Check identity and consent
6. Clean and drape
7. *Incision*: Long midline laparotomy
8. Prepare for rapid cannulation/perfusion
9. Warm phase dissection
10. Patient: 300 units/kg/body weight
11. Cannulation, perfusion and bleed out
12. While the perfusion is going on, collect spleen and lymph nodes for tissue matching/ HLA studies
13. Cold dissection
14. Close abdomen after swab count and instrument check.

15. In operation notes mention date and time of circulatory arrest clearly.

Donor Liver Harvest

While performing liver procurement, it is important to see if the liver is acceptable for donation and then do a proper donor hepatectomy and also reduce the warm ischemia time and the cold ischaemic time. Suitability of the donor liver is determined by visual inspection of an experienced liver transplant surgeon. After back table perfusion pack the liver in fresh HTK solution/UW solution in a plastic bowl into two bags sucking out air and place in ice box and ensure adequate ice is present.

Pancreas Procurement

The dissection of the pancreas is to be done very carefully to avoid damage to the blood supply of the liver and protect the pancreas. Visual inspection is an essential element to the pancreas procurement process. Once the organs have been adequately flushed, the liver and pancreas are either separated *in situ* and removed individually from the donor, or both organs are removed *en bloc* and divided at the back bench.

Intestinal Procurement

During procurement of a combined liver-intestine transplant, the liver, duodenum, pancreas, spleen, and small bowel are generally procured *en bloc*, thus avoiding any hilar dissection. For isolated Intestinal Transplantation, isolated intestine can be safely procured while still allowing for use of the liver and pancreas from the same donor.

Summary

Organized regional networks designed for the early identification of potential organ donors and rapid procurement in select candidates helps in the successful use of organ donation. As the recipient candidate having the end stage disease, these organ donations may be the only curative treatment option for thousands of patients. The role of the team leader and the donor coordinator are most important for successful outcome of organ donation.

Prevention of Liver Disease

Gaurav Mehta

INTRODUCTION

There are over 100 different forms of liver disease caused by a variety of factors ranging from viruses and genetics to toxins and poor nutrition. The good news is that many of the most common forms of liver disease can often be prevented by understanding risk factors, taking precautions and/or making healthy lifestyle choices. In the case of congenital liver disease, all that can be done is to treat symptoms as they arise. However, much can be done to prevent liver disease that is the result of a viral infection, or alcohol and drug abuse, or diet choices. Over time, damage to the liver results in scarring (cirrhosis), which can lead to liver failure, a life-threatening condition.

CAUSES OF LIVER DISEASE

Infection

Parasites and viruses can infect the liver, causing inflammation and that reduces liver function. The virus enters the blood through blood, semen, food, water and close contact. The most common types of liver infection are hepatitis viruses, including:
- Hepatitis A
- Hepatitis B
- Hepatitis C

Immune System Abnormality

Diseases in which your immune system attacks certain parts of your body (autoimmune) can affect your liver. Examples of autoimmune liver diseases include:
- Autoimmune hepatitis
- Primary biliary cirrhosis
- Primary sclerosing cholangitis

Genetics

An abnormal gene inherited from one or both of your parents can cause various substances to build up in your liver, resulting in liver damage. Genetic liver diseases include:
- Hemochromatosis
- Hyperoxaluria and oxalosis
- Wilson's disease

Cancer and Other Growths

Examples include
- Liver cancer
- Bile duct cancer
- Liver adenoma

Other

Additional, common causes of liver disease include
- Chronic alcohol abuse (Alcohol Liver Disease: ALD)
- Fat accumulating in the liver (non-alcoholic fatty liver disease)

PREVENTION

Prevention of liver disease is possible in many cases and the most important step that can be taken by patients and healthcare professionals. Here are some things that can be done to prevent liver disease caused by the above-mentioned things.

1. Maintaining a Healthy Weight

Fat accumulation in the liver because of an unhealthy diet can cause serious liver damage. It is known as non-alcoholic fatty liver disease (NAFLD & NASH) and often affects people who are overweight or obese. Weight loss is recommended, as are regular exercise and a healthy, low-fat, high fibre diet.

Some patients may require liver function tests, ultrasound and further testing. A smaller subset of these patients can require a liver biopsy depending on their clinical condition and risk factors for progressive disease. They also require follow-up visits with their gastroenterologist and hepatologist.

2. Excellent Hygiene

Good hygiene habits will go a long way to prevent hepatitis A & E. The virus is spread by coming into contact with infected faeces. It is essential to wash your hands after going to the toilet, and after changing a baby's nappy. You also need to wash your hands before working with food. Boil your drinking water if you are not sure that it is clean.

3. Vaccinations

You can be "vaccinated" against hepatitis by being given an injection that contains immuno-globulins or antibodies to the hepatitis A and B viruses. This is not effective if you have already been infected. Neonates are now vaccinated at birth for hepatitis B with a series of vaccination. A vaccine against hepatitis A is also available and is often used as a preventative mechanism for staff in day-care centres or in health settings.

4. Avoid Close Contact

Hepatitis B and C are blood-borne viruses. Hepatitis B is particularly infectious. Close contact (rough play amongst children, direct contact with the blood of an infected person, sharing of razors, unsterile tattooing instruments, sharing of needles among drug abusers, from mother to baby, unsafe sex) must be avoided in order to prevent infection with both hepatitis B and C.

5. Avoid paracetamol overdose

Paracetamol is the most frequently used over-the-counter painkiller. In western countries acetaminophen (paracetamol) overdose is the most common cause of liver failure. It is essential to stick to the recommended dosages of this medication, and not to take any medication without consulting your doctor. Medication and alcohol should never be mixed.

6. Over the Counter Health Supplements

Supplements and herbs, despite being "natural" can be toxic to the liver. There are a few natural products like chaparral, comfrey tea, skullcap, yohimbe, kava which can be toxic to liver. Weight loss products, excess of iron, vitamin A, alcohol, drugs, can lead to liver cirrhosis. Illegal drugs like heroin, cocaine, inhalants can cause liver damage.

7. Drink Moderately and Avoid Drug Use

Heavy drinking over a long period of time can cause inflammation in the liver. Scarring in the liver can lead to liver cirrhosis. The ability to process alcohol differs from person to person. According to the Dietary Guidelines for Americans, moderate alcohol consumption is defined as having up to 1 drink per day for women and up to 2 drinks per day for men. However, the Dietary Guidelines do not recommend that individuals who do not drink alcohol start drinking for any reason.

Illegal drugs such as heroin, cocaine and inhalants can cause severe liver injury and should be avoided at all costs.

Medication Use in People with Liver Disease

With very rare exceptions, when a patient with liver disease, e.g. hepatitis C, is given a drug (potentially toxic to the liver), the degree of damage would be higher than in a person with normal liver. Hence, care is taken to give only safe medication and some doctors avoid cholesterol reducing agents. This is done in spite of research showing that these medications are safely given in patients with fatty liver.

People with more severe types of liver disease such as cirrhosis have to be more careful regarding the types and dose of medications they take. The liver has a good ability to break down and use the medications even if the liver is severely damaged. Some medications should not be used or should be used at reduced dose when given to patients with advanced cirrhosis.

Recommendations to Minimize the Risk of Liver Injury from Medications

1. Always keep a list of all the prescription and non-prescription medications that you take, including herbs, vitamins and supplements. Bring this list with you to every physician's appointment.
2. The fewer medications you take the better. This includes herbs, supplements, prescription and non-prescription medications. If you are taking consultation from several doctors, be sure all of them are informed about your current list of medications.
3. When using non-prescription medications, be sure to read the label carefully and never exceed the recommended amount. However, the patient should avoid using the drug for prolonged period unless he consults his doctor.
4. If you are taking several medications, be sure the ingredients are not the same; otherwise you may risk taking an accidental overdose.
5. If you drink a significant amount of alcohol daily, avoid or restrict the use of acetaminophen; never take the maximum recommended dose.
6. If you have liver disease, make sure that your physician is aware of your diagnosis and the severity of your liver disease.
7. If you have advanced liver disease such as severe cirrhosis, it is a good idea to consult with the liver specialist before starting new medications.

3

Types of Liver Transplantation

Vikram Raut, Pathik Parikh, Darius Mirza

Liver transplantation is a definitive life-saving treatment for end stage liver disease. With improved surgical technique and immuno-suppression, 1-year survival after liver transplantation is approximately 90% in high volume centres. Donor availability is the principal limiting factor for expansion of liver transplantation. This chapter aims to address the different types of liver transplantation procedure.

ORTHOTOPIC LIVER TRANSPLANTATION (OLT)

The most commonly used technique of liver transplantation is orthotopic transplantation, in which native liver is removed and replaced by the donor organ in the same anatomic location as the original liver.

Deceased Donor Liver Transplantation

In this type of liver transplantation, the donor organ comes from a deceased donor—an

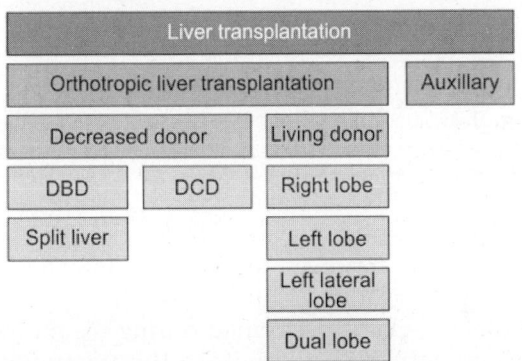

Fig. 3.1: Types of liver transplantation

individual from whom at least one solid organ is recovered for the purpose of transplantation after suffering brain or cardiac death.

DONATION AFTER BRAIN DEATH (DBD)

These were formally called heart-beating donors and are derived from patients who have suffered brain stem death. These are intensive care unit-based patients with apnoeic coma of known cause, most cases of brain stem death are caused by trauma or intracerebral haemorrhage. In these donors, the heart is beating and the intra-thoracic and intra-abdominal organs are perfuse with oxygenated blood right up to the point of procurement. Therefore, there is little warm ischemic injury to the organs prior to retrieval. Due to the shortage of donor organs to meet the growing demand, transplantation from an expanded criteria donor may also be an option for some transplant candidates.

Traditionally, liver transplantation in adult patients has been performed using the conventional caval reconstruction technique with veno-venous bypass (Fig. 3.2a). Conventional technique involves recipient hepatectomy including the retrohepatic vena cava. Conventional technique has been a reliable and standard technique. However, hypotension due to the clamping of the major vessels, bleeding from the retroperitoneum, longer vascular reconstruction time, and

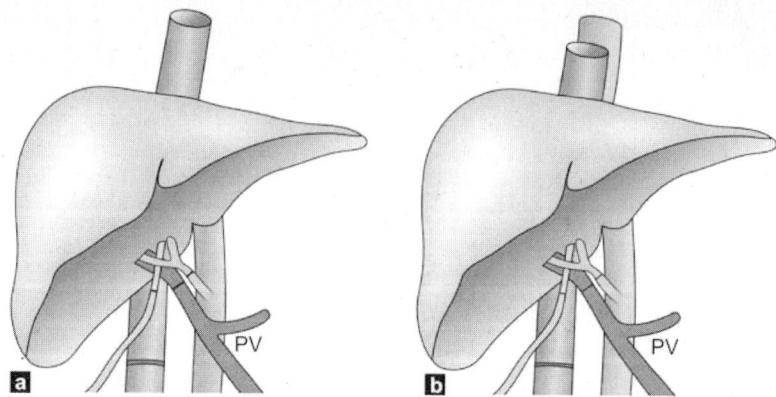

Fig. 3.2: Techniques of orthotropic liver transplantation: (a) Conventional caval replacement; (b) piggyback technique

complication of veno-venous bypass have been the shortcomings of conventional technique. Recently, the advantages of piggyback technique have been reported, including lower amount of usage of blood products, shorter operating time, and declining use of veno-venous bypass. Piggyback technique involves hepatectomy with preservation of native retrohepatic vena cava (Fig. 3.2b). Piggyback technique also has a few shortcomings, which include outflow obstruction, specifically in the hepatic venous cuff anastomosis.

Split Liver Transplantation

Paediatric liver transplantation has driven technical innovations in surgery over the past 25 years. Early successful liver transplantation relied on the use of size-matched whole-liver grafts. This requirement tended to exclude small children of less than 10 kg from liver transplantation because of the lack of donors. Reduction techniques based on the segmental anatomy of the liver were developed to reduce waiting list mortality and transplant smaller children. Liver reduction proved to be successful; however, it led to the discarding of the right liver with a fall in the number of grafts from young donors available for adult recipients. The concept of "splitting" one liver for two recipients was developed to use both lobes and is now an established technique associated with excellent outcomes (Fig. 3.3).

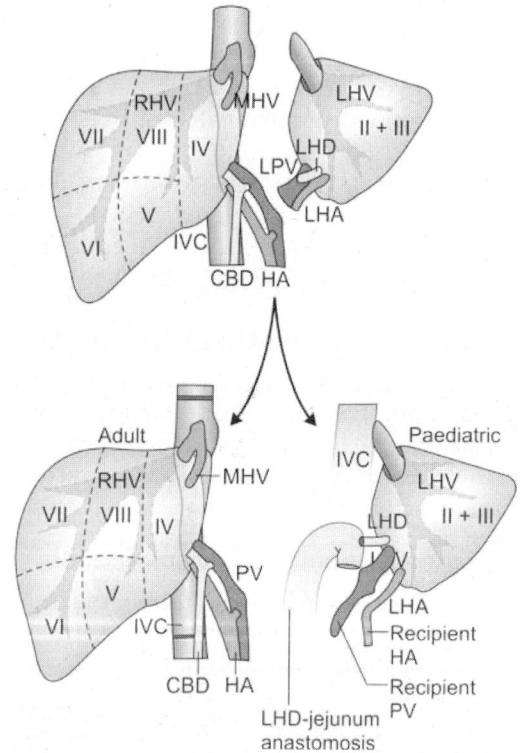

Fig. 3.3: Liver graft is split into two grafts, left lateral segment used for paediatric liver transplantation and rest of graft used for adult recipient

Ex situ splitting is performed after the donor liver has been retrieved and perfused with preservation solution.

In situ split is performed during the multi-organ retrieval and before the perfusion with preservation solution. The donor liver parenchyma is divided while maintaining an intact blood supply through the left lateral segment.

DONATION AFTER CARDIAC DEATH (DCD)

Over the past 15 years, as the shortage of organs for transplantation has become more severe, there has been an increasing emphasis on DCD. After consent for organ donation is obtained, the patient is brought to the operating room, life support is withdrawn, and when the heart stops after a few minutes to an hour without ventilation or other support, the physician observes the patient for a few minutes to ensure that the heart does not start beating again spontaneously. If there continues to be no circulation for 2–5 minutes, the physician pronounces the patient dead. At this point, the transplant team enters the operating room and removes organs, usually the kidneys and liver, from the now dead patient.

LIVING DONOR LIVER TRANSPLANTATION (LDLT)

An increase in the number of people awaiting liver transplantation, many of whom cannot survive the waiting time for a deceased donor organ, has led more patients and their families to explore the option of LDLT. In this procedure a healthy, living person donates a portion of liver to recipient. In addition to less waiting time to transplantation, LDLT also provides improved graft and patient survival rates and gives the flexibility of scheduling surgery.

When considering LDLT, it is important to consider the need for an adequately sized graft for the recipient with sufficient residual mass for the donor. Outcomes are better with a graft-to-recipient body weight ratio greater than 0.8%.

Right Lobe Living Donor Liver Transplantation

Right lobe LDLT overcomes the restriction imposed by donor-recipient size matching and is the main workload in centres active in adult LDLT. Adult right liver LDLT is a complicated and technically demanding procedure. The middle hepatic vein serves as an important landmark for the plane of the transection within the liver parenchyma. In recipient operation right hepatic vein and middle hepatic vein or reconstructed middle hepatic vein is anastomosed to IVC in the recipient (Fig. 3.4).

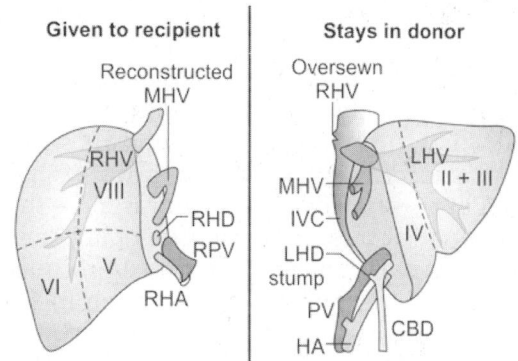

Fig. 3.4: Right lobe living donor liver transplantation, right lobe graft consists of right hepatic vein (RHV), reconstructed middle hepatic vein (MHV), right hepatic artery (RHA), right portal vein (RPV) and right hepatic duct (RHD)

Left Lobe Living Donor Liver Transplantation

A left liver graft may be a safer alternative to a right liver graft for donors, and they are now used for properly selected cases in several centres. The left lobe graft has the left and middle hepatic arteries, left portal vein, left bile duct and left and middle hepatic vein. Parenchymal transection is performed along the right side of the middle hepatic vein. In recipient operation the left and middle hepatic veins of the recipient are anastomosed with the graft vein (Fig. 3.5).

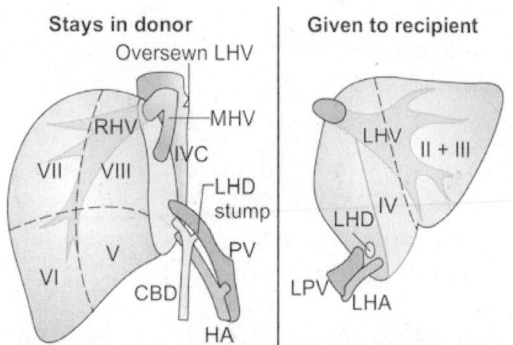

Fig. 3.5: Left lobe living donor liver transplantation, left lobe graft consists of left hepatic vein (LHV), left hepatic artery (LHA), left portal vein (LPV) and left hepatic duct (LHD)

Left Lateral Living Donor Liver Transplantation

Left lateral segment grafts are most commonly used in children (Fig. 3.6). In smaller children the partial or reduced left lateral segment (segment II or segment III, or reduced both). Selection of the graft is based on the potential volume of the graft in relation to the recipient's body size. Graft recipient weight ratio is within 1% to 3%, the graft size is considered adequate. If the ratio of graft weight to recipient body weight is more than 4%, poor perfusion of the graft may cause unsatisfactory primary function. In recipient surgery, left hepatic vein is anastomosed with triangular hepatic veins—IVC opening. Interrupted suture is recommended in patients with a small portal vein. Reconstruction of the dominant artery may be sufficient without reconstructing other arteries in patients with multiple arterial supply to the graft.

Dual-lobe Liver Transplantation

For adult LDLT, insufficient graft size has been a major obstacle. At the same time, the safety of donors must have top priority when considering LDLT. A donor with right lobe volume >70% of total liver volume on preoperative volumetric computed tomography should not be allowed to donate the right lobe. As an alternative, dual left lobe or left lateral segment transplantation can be an option to avoid the small-for-size-graft problem caused by a left lobe liver transplantation alone when the critical right lobectomy poses an independent donor risk.

A right lobe and left lobe dual-graft transplantation from two independent donors can be performed to a large-size recipient to avoid the small-for-size-graft problem (Fig. 3.7).

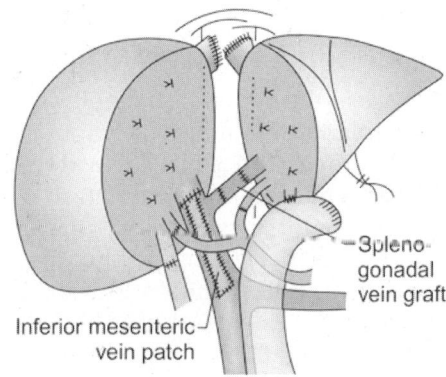

Inferior mesenteric vein patch

Spleno-gonadal vein graft

Fig. 3.7: Right lobe and left lobe dual-graft transplantation

Auxiliary Liver Transplantation

Auxiliary transplantation uses a partial left or right lobe from the donor which acts as temporary support for the recipient's injured liver, which remains in place (Fig. 3.8). Once the native liver recovers, immunosuppression is withdrawn and the graft is either surgically removed or is allowed to atrophy naturally. The partial graft is placed below the native liver (heterotopic auxiliary transplantation) or replaces the resected right or left native lobe (auxiliary partial liver transplantation). The best outcomes with auxiliary transplantation are in young patients with hyperacute presentations.

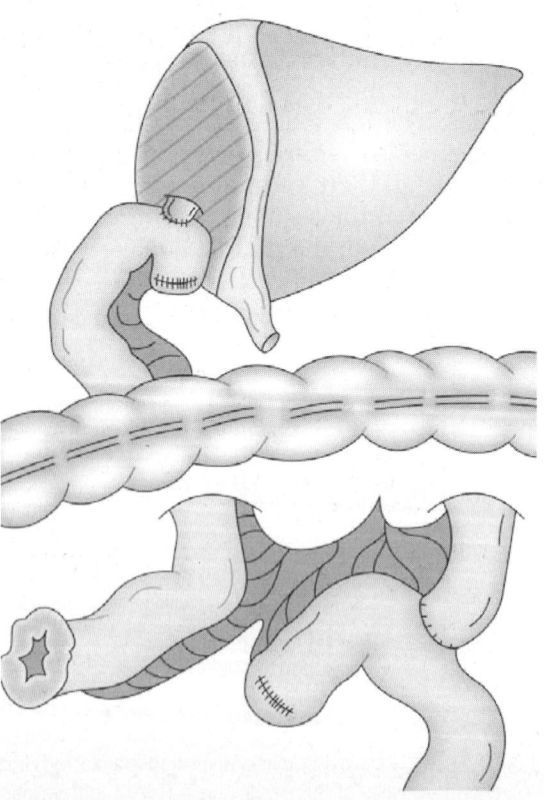

Fig. 3.6: Left lateral living donor liver transplantation

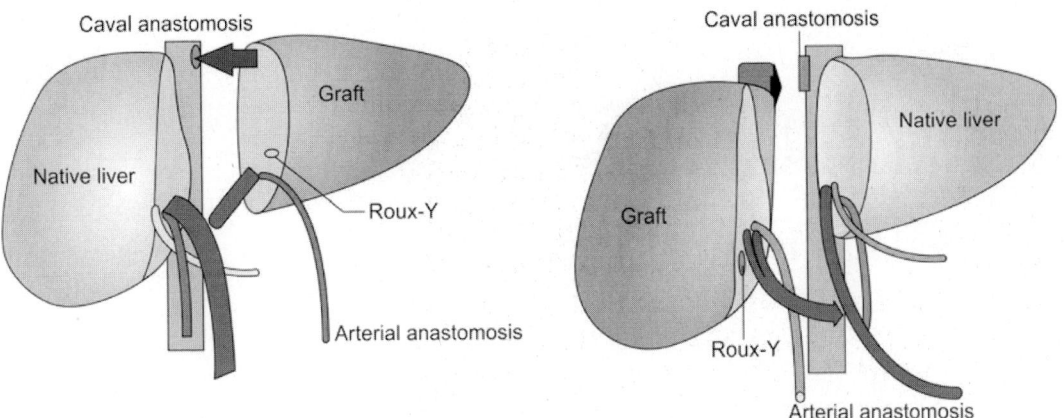

Fig. 3.8: Auxiliary liver transplantation

Pre-transplant Medical Evaluation of Liver Transplant Recipient

Ankur Shah

INTRODUCTION

Liver transplantation is a physically and emotionally challenging endeavour that is stressful to patients and their families. A thorough and detailed evaluation is therefore necessary. The goal of the workup is fourfold:

1. It must establish a diagnosis of chronic liver disease, the severity of the disease and the possible cause
2. It must exclude any absolute or relative contraindication to the liver transplant surgery
3. The patient is in a relatively stable physical and mental health to undergo a long and complex surgery
4. Finally, it must assess the suitability of each patient to better allocate a cadaveric organ and optimize survival (irrespective of a living or cadaveric donor).

The pre-transplant medical workup includes

- A detailed history
- Clinical examination
- Variety of laboratory and radiological tests.

History

- Current symptoms related to underlying liver disease and other comorbid medical condition
- Detailed past history of any cardiac (heart), pulmonary (chest) issues or any cancers
- Full evaluation of the candidate's past, present, and future risk of exposure to infection including tuberculosis

- A complete vaccination history
- Current medications and allergies.
- Drug and alcohol abuse
- Social history (especially for transplant co-ordinators as it is an excellent opportunity to engage household members and other close contacts in the education and protection of the future recipient).

Clinical Examination

A thorough general and systemic examination is performed to specifically look for the following

- Signs of chronic liver disease
- Any potential cardiac/respiratory or neurological issue
- Nutritional status including malnutrition or obesity
- Focus of infection

Laboratory and radiology tests
Blood tests
1 ABO blood grouping + Rh typing
2 Complete blood count with peripheral smear
3 Liver function test
4 Renal function test
5 Magnesium
6 Glucose fasting/post prandial
7 Glycosylated haemoglobin (HbA1c)
8 Prothrombin time/international normalised ratio (PT/INR)
9 Activated partial thromboplastin time (APTT)

10 Fibrinogen
11 Lipid profile
12 Thyroid profile
13 Ferritin

Tumour markers

14 AFP (alpha fetoprotein)
15 CEA (carcinoembryonic antigen)
16 CA19.9 (cancer antigen 19-9)
17 CA 125 (females)
18 PSA (Males)

Viral Markers

19 CMV IgG/IgM (cytomegalovirus)
20 HbsAg (hepatitis B surface antigen) antiHbe/ HbeAg/HBV DNA viral load
21 Anti Hbc-total (hepatitis B core antibody)
22 Anti HBs antibodies
23 Anti HCV (hepatitis C virus)
24 HIV I-II (human immunodeficiency virus)
25 VDRL (venereal disease research laboratory test)

Cultures

26 Urine
27 Blood
28 Ascitic fluid culture
29 Sputum
30 Urine RE/ME (routine examination/microscopic examination)
31 24 hours urine protein creatinine ratio
32 24 hours urine creatinine clearance

Pulmonary evaluation

33 HRCT chest (high resolution computed tomography)
34 Pulmonary function test (PFT)
35 Arterial blood gas (ABG)
36 Arterial lactate
37 Pleural fluid culture

Cardiac evaluation

38 ECG (electrocardiography)
39 2D echo
40 Dobutamine stress echo (angiography in select cases)

Radiology

41 Ultrasonography abdomen
42 Contrast enhanced computed tomography (CECT) triple phase of abdomen

Additional test for females (if required)

43 UPT (urine pregnancy test)
44 Ultrasonography pelvis
45 Pap smear
46 Mammography/sonomammography

Besides the above, an upper gastro-intestinal endoscopy (OGD) is performed on all potential recipients.

Once, all the reports are available, mandatory consultations and clearances from the following specialities are needed:
• Hepatologist (liver physician)
• Transplant surgeon
• Cardiologist
• Pulmonary physician
• Psychiatrist
• Dentist
• Anaesthetist
• Dietician
• Physiotherapist
• Gynaecologist (for female recipients)
• Financial clearance

Once the workup is complete, all workup results and consultations are presented at the Liver Transplant Clinical meeting. This meeting is generally attended by:
• Transplant surgeons
• Hepatologists
• Anaesthetist
• Intensivist
• Pathologist
• Radiologist
• Transplant co-ordinator
• Primary care physician (if possible).

The work-up and structure of the committee may vary slightly with different centres, however, the process is uniform and primarily involves answering the following questions.
• Does the patient need liver transplant as therapy for his or her disease?
• Have the indications and contraindications been properly assessed?
• What is the surgical risk and prognosis?
• Is the patient's medical condition such that he or she will be able to tolerate the procedure and postoperative course?

• What are the chances of recurrent disease affecting graft and patient survival?

Patients are excluded if they were too well, too sick, too old or had other comorbid conditions (e.g. severe heart disease), substance abuse problems (e.g. not abstinent from alcohol intake), or any other psychosocial barriers that may not augur well for the survival of the graft.

Once candidates have undergone routine screening, an individualized approach is warranted to identify particular predisposing factors that may predict infection/risk factors and outcome. Assessment may need to be periodically repeated in patients who remain on the cadaveric waiting list, with 6 monthly investigations and viral screening as the preferred standard in most centres, and more frequent testing if indicated.

The key to successful pre-transplant evaluation is the recognition of risk, the acquisition of information, a multi-disciplinary team decision that would result in an organized and thoughtful approach to perioperative and post-transplant management, thus ensuring best outcomes.

Post-liver Transplant Medication and Precaution

Jayshri Shah

INTRODUCTION

The goal of transplantation is not only to ensure survival of patients but also to offer patients the opportunity to achieve a good balance between the functional efficacy of the graft and their physical and psychological well-being. Patient usually remains in hospital for 2–3 weeks after a transplant. Following discharge it is important to follow the instructions to ensure a good outcome.

The long-term success of any transplant depends on numerous factors:

1. Regular review with transplant team following their advice, including performing the laboratory tests and monitoring protocol. Initially the visits are frequent, once in few days then once in 2 weeks. Usually after the first year, frequency of follow-up is reduced to once in 3 months. Also the frequency of monitoring drug immunosuppression levels is high in first year of transplantation and reduced to once every 3 months after the first year.
2. Taking the medication as prescribed in correct doses and interval to avoid the organ from rejection. Most patients will receive a combination of three anti-rejection medication including tacrolimus/cyclosporine, azathioprine/mycophenolate and prednisolone (depending on centre preference) post-transplant in the first three months. Due to higher doses of immunosuppressive medication, the patient is at risk of opportunistic infections and therefore will be on number of prophylactic medications including antibiotics, antifungal, antiviral medication in the first 3 months after transplant. Steroids are usually tapered off over 3–6 months and doses of other immunosuppressive drugs is also gradually reduced over the first year. Most post-transplant patients will be left with only one or two anti-rejection medication after 1 year of transplantation.
3. To follow some precautions in view of long-term immmnosuppressive medication.

Precautions to be Taken after a Liver Transplant

Eating: Avoid eating outside food and on the road-side. Boil your drinking water. Wash fruits and vegetables thoroughly before consumption. Wash your hands before eating.

Exercise: Avoid strenuous physical activity for 6 weeks after a transplant. Light physical activity helps to improve physical and mental well-being. Avoid swimming and outdoor sports until the incision has healed. During exercise if you experience any chest pain, shortness of breath or light headedness, you should stop your workout immediately and see the doctor. 15–20 mins of walking daily is recommended and gradually increase as tolerated.

Driving: This is prohibited for at least 4–6 weeks after a transplant and may be longer as some of the medication used after transplant can reduce your alertness level, cause tremors and blurring of vision.

Smoking: Smoking is harmful to health due to multiple side-effects including risk of lung, oral and gastrointestinal tract cancers. Also, smoking increases the risk of hypertension. All post-transplant patients should be encouraged to avoid smoking and assistance should be provided to achieve that goal.

Alcohol: Combining alcohol with anti-rejection medication may harm the liver. All post-transplant patients should be advised to avoid alcohol as it is independent risk factor for liver damage.

Medical alert: It is important for all transplant patients to wear a medical alert identification bracelet. Always keep all documents regarding medical history and current medication at all times.

Return to school or work: After a transplant one can return to school or work within 2–3 months after discussion with the transplant team. Initially post-transplant patient has less energy, as it takes time for the body to heal and adjust to new medication.

Travel: Within first 2–3 months after transplant is not recommended. Travel outside the continent is prohibited for 6–12 months after transplant due to the concern regarding vaccines and lack of immunity to infections unique to various continents.

Pets: Many patients may have pets and would be concerned regarding risk of transmission of infections in view of anti-rejection medication, it is best to avoid them:

- Cats are fine, but the transplant recipient should avoid changing the litter box as toxoplasmosis is spread to people through cat feces.

- Dogs are permitted as long as they have regular check-ups and vaccination.

- Avoid fish as the aquarium water can spread unusual infections specially through cuts and sores on a recipients hand.

- Birds are not permitted, as they carry diseases which are transmitted to people.

Routine Self-examination and Health Maintenance

- *De novo* malignancy is one of the leading causes of mortality after liver transplantation.

- The risk of skin cancer and lymphoma are more than ten fold greater than the risk in age-matched and sex-matched general population.

- Developing certain cancers such as lung, head, neck and colorectal neoplasia is more common when taking immunosuppressive medication. Due to this, monthly breast and testicular self-examination is recommended. PAP smear, breast exams, testicular exams, skin cancer screening should be done annually.

Immunizations and Vaccinations

- Post-transplantation, only dead virus vaccines are allowed after 1 year.

- Live virus vaccines such as varicella, MMR are contraindicated because of risk of transmission

- Care must be taken once in contact with family members who are recently immunized, especially infants receiving the polio vaccine, as the virus will be shed in the stool.

Skin Care

- Post-transplant patients are prone to acne due to immunosuppressive medication such as prednisolone and cyclosporine

- Cuts, scratches, dry skin should be treated to prevent infections

- *Sun exposure*: Immunosupressive medication increases risk of skin and lip cancers. Prednisolone makes your skin more sensitive to the sun. Prolonged and repeated exposure to sun produces permanent and damaging skin changes.

- Avoiding sun exposure and using UV protection sun cream is recommended

Hair Care

- Anti-rejection medication such as prednisolone, tacrolimus can cause excess hair loss.

- Prednisolone and cyclosporine can cause excessive hair growth which can be a troublesome side-effect for women. Standard hair removal creams can be used.

Dental Care

- All patients have a pre-transplant dental assessment.
- Routine dental work can be done 6 months post-transplant.
- Post-transplant, it is important to take an antibiotic before any dental work including polishing and cleaning.
- It is important to maintain good oral hygiene and brushing your teeth twice a day.
- Dental flossing is good for overall dental hygiene, but flossing can irritate your gums and cause bleeding, so this should be done gently.

Eye Care

It is important to have annual eye check up with ophthalmologist as immunosuppressant medication particularly prednisolone increases risk of cataract formation. First post-transplant eye assessment should be done at 6 months and then annually.

Sexual activity: Sexual dysfunction and sex hormone disturbances are widely reported in men and women with chronic liver disease before liver transplant. Sexual dysfunction is characterized by disturbances in sexual desire and in psychophysiological changes associated with sexual response cycle in men and women. Although successful liver transplant should lead to improvement in sexual function, immunosuppressive drugs may interfere with hormone metabolism.

- Women usually return to regular menstrual cycle within 2–3 months post-transplant. Ovulation may take place before regular menstrual cycle, therefore birth control measures should be used to avoid conception for up to 1 yr after transplantation. Barrier contraception appears to be the safest option.
- In men erectile dysfunction has been reported in 10–50% with chronic liver disease. Although some improvement in number of sexual function is reported after

liver transplant, in a proportion of men the erectile dysfunction persists. The risk is increased with age, smoking, alcohol, diabetes and concomitant medication for depression, hypertension.

- **Immunosuppressive drugs and gonadal dysfunction:** There has been a link between use of sirolimus and decreased spermatogenesis in some studies.

Pregnancy

- Pregnancy should be avoided for 12 months after a transplant.
- Pregnancy is often successful after liver transplant despite potentially toxic effects of immunosuppressive medication.
- There is no increase in the risk of graft rejection during pregnancy.
- Liver transplant recipients with recurrent hepatitis C or B appear to be at risk of worse graft function in event of pregnancy and some of antiviral medication is contraindicated in pregnancy due to the teratogenic effects.
- *Immunosuppressive drugs and pregnancy:* The immunosuppressive medication should be continued during pregnancy to avoid graft rejection and it is important to monitor the drug concentration periodically. It is preferred to maintain the pregnant patient on single immunosuppressive drug regimen such as tacrolimus or cyclosporine. Cyclosporine, tacrolimus and sirolimus have been considered Class C drugs in terms of its risk for pregnancy by the FDA. Corticosteroids is considered class B drug. Both azathioprine and mycophenolate mofetil have been classified as Class D drugs, although use of azathioprine after first trimester has been considered relatively safe.
- *Fetal outcome:* Fetal loss, prematurity and low birth weight have been reported in women who have undergone transplantation.
- *Maternal outcome:* The maternal risks include hypertension, pre-eclampsia, gestational diabetes and graft dysfunction. The rate of caesarean section is considerably higher in post-transplant patients. It is

important for post-transplant patients who conceive to be managed in centres with multidisciplinary teams including transplant physician, obstetrician and pediatrician.

- *Immunosuppressive drugs and breast feeding:* Most transplant centres advise against breast feeding because of concerns over safety of neonatal exposure to immuno-suppressive drugs, corticosteroids, cyclosporine and tacrolimus are excreted in breast milk, whereas no data reported for sirolimus.

Risk of Comorbidities after Transplantation

The most common causes of death beyond the first year of transplant are (in descending order of frequency) graft failure, malignancy, cardiovascular disease, infections and renal failure:

- Chronic kidney disease is a common complication after liver transplantation and has major impact on graft survival. This is usually due to immunosuppressive drugs such as cyclosporine and tacrolimus (calcineurin inhibitor toxicity). Regular follow-up with transplant physician is therefore recommended so that the medication can be altered to minimize the toxicity.
- **Metabolic syndrome and cardiovascular disease:** There is a high prevalence of cardiovascular risk factors such as hypertension, obesity, diabetes, dyslipidemia (metabolic syndrome) in transplant recipients. This results in increasing incidence of premature onset of cardiovascular disease,

which is three times higher compared to general population. It is therefore important to emphasize healthy lifestyle including balanced diet and regular exercise to help with control of the cardiovascular risk factors along with appropriate medication.

Summary

Survival after transplantation continues to improve with newer anti-rejection medication. However, the use of immunosuppressive medicines increases the risk of developing obesity, dyslipidemia, diabetes, hypertension and metabolic syndrome, thereby contributing to increased cardiovascular risk. Also use of immunosuppressants increases risk of infections, skin disorders, metabolic bone disease and malignancies.

Following the regular monitoring protocol, follow-up with transplant centre and using adequate precautions including healthy life-style will help early recognition and aggressive risk factor modification which should translate into improved long-term outcomes after transplantation.

Further Reading

1. Liver transplantation: Volume 15, Number 11, Supplement 2, November 2009.
2. Liver transplantation: Volume 18, Number 11, Supplement 2, November 2013.
3. Medical care of the transplant patient, 4th Edition, Clavien and Trotter.

Anatomy and Physiology of the Bowel

Vinay Kumaran

The intestines (or gut) are the main organ of digestion and absorption of nutrition in our body. The 'small intestine' extends from the duodenum, into which the stomach opens, to the caecum, which is the beginning of the 'large intestine'. The large intestine extends from the caecum to the anus.

Anatomy of the Bowels

The duodenum is the C-shaped initial part of the small bowel which begins where the pylorus of the stomach ends. The sphincter of the pylorus keeps food in the stomach and releases it slowly into the duodenum by periodically relaxing. The duodenum also receives the openings of the bile duct and the pancreatic duct. The duodenum shares its blood supply with the pancreas and, for all practical purposes, surgically needs to be treated as a unit with the head of the pancreas. It is included with the pancreas when doing a pancreas transplant.

The duodenum opens into the jejunum which is the upper (or proximal) part of the small intestine. The jejunum, imperceptibly transitions into the ileum. The jejunum and ileum together form the small bowel. Although different somewhat in function, there is no clear anatomical demarcation between the jejunum and the ileum. There is a gradual transition from the jejunum to the ileum. The jejunum secretes enzymes and a lot of the digestion of food happens here. Most of the absorption of food and vitamins as well as bile salts occurs in the ileum. The last 2 feet of the ileum is particularly important for absorption of vitamin B_{12} and bile salts. The small intestine is normally about 6 meters in length of which the ileum is the longer part.

The ileum opens into the beginning of the large intestine, the caecum. The junction of the ileum and the caecum has a valve which is a common site for intestinal tuberculosis. The appendix is a blind tubular structure which opens into the caecum. The wall of the appendix has a lot of lymphatic tissue. The appendix is prone to getting infected (appendicitis) and this infection can be dangerous if not managed in a timely fashion. The appendix can be safely removed in humans as it does not seem to do anything useful. In some animals, the appendix is much larger and helps in digestion.

The ascending colon lies on the right side of the abdomen. It is relatively thin walled and is a common site for cancer as well as amoebiasis. The transverse mesocolon extends across the upper part of the abdomen and is close to the gall bladder, the liver, the duodenum, and the stomach. On the left, it is close to the spleen. The right side of the transverse colon is called the hepatic flexure and the left side is called the splenic flexure.

The descending colon lies on the left side of the abdomen. It is more thick walled. The colon absorbs most of the water from the undigestible bowel content which reaches it and the descending colon contains largely solid faecal matter. Since the descending colon is relatively narrower than the ascending colon, cancers here tend to cause obstruction relatively early.

The descending colon opens into a relatively mobile part of the colon called the sigmoid flexure. This tends to be longer in vegetarians who have more fibre in their diet and may occasionally be so long that it can get twisted around itself (sigmoid volvulus) or around a loop of ileum (ileosigmoid knotting).

The sigmoid flexure opens into the rectum which is a wider part of the GI tract which lies in the pelvis. The rectum has large enough capacity to serve as a reservoir, allowing us to postpone defecation until it is convenient. The rectum is also a common site for cancer. Haemorrhoids (piles) are masses of soft tissue with dilated veins in the wall of the rectum. They are prone to bleed or even prolapse (protrude outside the anus).

The anal canal is the passage from the rectum to the opening of the anus. It is surrounded by the muscles of the anal sphincter which give us control over defecation. Unlike the rectum which is sensitive only to stretching, the lining of the anal canal does have touch and pain sensation. Infection of the glands near the anus can produce very painful perianal abscesses. An abscess eventually bursts either into the skin (sometimes forming a sinus) or into the anal canal or rectum, discharging the pus within and giving relief from the pain. An abscess which opens both into the perianal skin and into the anus or rectum forms a track called a fistula. A fistula tends to get infected repeatedly.

Indications for Intestinal Transplant

Like other organs, the intestine can fail. Its functions are to digest and absorb food and to expel the undigested portion of the food. One reason for intestinal failure, of course, is if the intestine needs to be removed. The commonest cause for having to remove the intestine is when blockage of the blood vessels to the intestine leads to gangrene.

There are several blood vessels which supply blood to the intestine. The duodenum receives blood from branches of the celiac axis. The jejunum, ileum, caecum, ascending colon and the right two-thirds of the transverse colon get blood from the superior mesenteric artery. The left one-third of the transverse colon, the descending colon and the upper part of the rectum get blood from the inferior mesenteric artery. The lower part of the rectum and the anal canal get blood from branches of the internal iliac artery. Normally there are communications between the arterial branches and blockage of any one artery is unlikely to cause gangrene of the entire bowel. However, sometimes the adjacent arteries are also narrowed by atherosclerosis and blockage of an artery can lead to extensive gangrene.

We can manage without the large intestine at the cost of more frequent and more liquid stools but the small intestine is essential for life. After removal of part of the intestine, the rest of the intestine does adapt. It becomes larger, the villi (folds in the lining) increase in number to increase the surface area and so on. However, there is a limit to the adaptation and it is estimated that if less than 60 cm of small bowel is left, the patient will be dependent on intravenous (parenteral) nutrition.

Total Parenteral Nutrition (TPN) can keep a patient with intestinal failure alive, theoretically for long periods of time but there are problems with TPN. TPN has to be administered via a central venous catheter (CVC). The presence of the catheter eventually causes clotting (thrombosis) of the vein and the catheter stops working. It must be removed and another catheter placed in another vein. Eventually it becomes increasingly difficult to find a vein. Another risk of a central venous catheter is the risk of infection in the blood stream which can be life-threatening. An infected CVC needs to be removed and a new one placed in a different vein.

Over a period, TPN can affect the liver, which becomes first fatty, then cholestatic (retaining bilirubin) and eventually scarred and cirrhotic. Worsening liver function is an indication for intestinal transplantation. If the transplant is delayed too much then the patient may require transplantation of the liver as well as the intestine.

Other reasons for removal of the intestine include Crohn's disease which a form of inflammatory bowel disease in which the intestine becomes scarred and obstructed. Repeated operations for intestinal obstruction result in removing more and more of the intestine until the patient is TPN dependent. Desmoid tumours are slowly growing, locally invasive tumours which can grow around the root of the mesentery (from where the blood vessels reach the intestines) and removing these tumours may require removal of most or all the small intestine.

There is a group of disorders called intestinal motility disorders in which the normal propulsive contractions in the wall of the intestine are lost. The result is similar to intestinal obstruction and the only long-term treatment when surgical and medical measures are exhausted may be an intestinal transplant.

Summary

1. The intestines are vital life-sustaining organs without which we cannot survive.
2. They have considerable reserve and capacity to adapt but when the reserve is exhausted, transplantation may be the only option to save the patient's life.

Treatment and Transplant of Intestine

Hunaid Hatimi, Somnath Chattopadhyay, Ravi Mohanka

INTRODUCTION

Bowel (intestinal) transplantation is performed to replace a diseased or shortened small bowel with healthy bowel typically from a deceased (cadaveric) donor. Intestinal transplant helps avoid life-threatening complications of peripheral nutrition, improves the quality of life and increased longevity.

Indications

Intestinal failure is defined as an inability to maintain sufficient electrolyte, nutrient, and fluid balance for more than 1 month without total parenteral nutrition (TPN) with no adaptive potential.

In certain situations, patients may require massive resection of intestine as a life-saving measure, generally due to gangrene. However, it results in short-bowel syndrome, inability to digest food and diarrhoea. This situation may also arise in certain diseases in children and adults, where although the length of the intestine may be normal, its function is affected. Currently, such patients are managed by giving TPN, which ensures adequate nutrition. However, TPN is associated with complications in the long term, commonly due to long-term central line usage. Patients who are facing difficulties with TPN are candidates for intestinal transplantation.

Failure of TPN is defined as

- Impending or overt liver failure due to TPN-induced liver injury

- Thrombosis of two or more central veins
- Two or more episodes per year of catheter-related systemic sepsis that requires hospitalization
- A single episode of line-related fungemia, septic shock, or acute respiratory distress syndrome
- Frequent episodes of severe dehydration despite intravenous fluid supplementation in addition to TPN

Identifying and listing patients for intestinal transplant before liver dysfunction sets in, is important as it affects the survival (1-year survival 42% vs. 80% without transplant) and the need for small intestine alone vs liver-intestine transplant. Some of the common causes of intestinal failure in children and adults are as follows:

Children	Adults
Intestinal atresia	Crohn's disease
Gastroschisis	Superior mesenteric artery thrombosis
Crohn's disease	Superior mesenteric vein thrombosis
Microvillus involution disease	Trauma
Necrotizing enterocolitis	Desmoid tumor
Midgut volvulus (leading to infarction)	Volvulus
Chronic intestinal pseudo-obstruction	Pseudo-obstruction
Massive resection secondary to tumor	Massive resection secondary to tumor
Hirschsprung's disease	Radiation enteritis

Contraindications

The contraindications for intestinal transplant are essentially the same as is seen in other types of transplants. Examples include the following:

- Significant coexistent medical conditions
- An active uncontrolled infection or malignancy
- Psychosocial factors (e.g. the lack of capability to assume the responsibilities of the day-to-day management following the transplant or the absence of family support)

Types

There are three main types of intestinal transplants.

Isolated Intestinal Transplant

In this procedure, the affected portion of the small intestine is removed and replaced with healthy small intestine. It is suitable for patients with intestinal failure (shortening or dysfunction) only, without any liver dysfunction.

Liver-Intestine Transplantation

This procedure is performed for patients with intestinal failure and moderate to severe liver failure. It can also be performed for patients with liver failure or liver cirrhosis and extensive porto-mesenteric thrombosis, where a liver transplant alone may not be technically feasible. In this procedure, the patient's liver is removed along with the affected intestine and replaced with healthy block of liver and small intestine from the donor. The liver also offers some protection to the intestine against rejection.

Multi-visceral Transplantation

In certain diseases, not only the small and large intestines are affected, the stomach is also affected with motility disorder. In some large or aggressive tumors or trauma, resection may involve all the organs. In such patients, in addition to the liver and intestine, stomach, duodenum and pancreas are also transplanted, as a single cluster of organs, and is called a multi-visceral transplant. It involves removing the patient's liver and intestine and transplanting a cluster of organs from the donor (the patient's own pancreas and spleen are typically not removed).

Pre-transplant Recipient Evaluation

Transplant evaluation is performed by a multi-disciplinary team which includes a transplant surgeon, hepatologist, gastro-enterologist, anaesthesiologist, intensivist, cardiologist, infectious disease specialist, social worker, pharmacist, dietician, psychologist and others and involves the following:

- Patient's past medical and surgical records, prior endoscopic and radiologic evaluations are reviewed in detail. Motility studies (specially for stomach and large intestine) may be required.
- Blood grouping and human leukocyte antigen (HLA) typing is performed for cross-matching.
- Ultrasound of the liver and central veins is obtained to assess the vasculature.
- A liver biopsy is done in patients with suspected liver disease, although it may not be required in those with obvious clinical features of advanced liver disease.
- Serological studies include testing for human immune deficiency virus (HIV), hepatitis B virus, and hepatitis C virus, cytomegalovirus, Epstein-Barr virus.
- In patients with history of mesenteric vessel thrombosis, hypercoagulable evaluation is done.

The aim of evaluation is to determine the type of surgery required, fitness for surgery and the urgency of the operation.

Donor Selection

Criteria for selecting cadaveric donors are as follows:

- Younger donors <40 years are preferred.
- Donors smaller than the recipient, i.e. about 50% to 75% the size of the recipient are preferred, as these patients may have a small abdominal cavity and the organs may not fit easily.
- There should be no previous history of significant intestinal disease.
- The donors should be stable with no significant hemodynamic instability, sepsis,

history of malignancy or chronic infection, severe hypoxia or acidosis.

- Cold ischemia time should be <6 hours, therefore mostly organs from local donors are preferred.

Organ Retrieval

The donor surgery is like procurement of the liver and pancreas retrieval using a long midline incision. Vascular anatomy of the liver, size match of the organs for the recipient are important considerations and should be discussed between the donor and recipient teams before finalizing the retrieval plan. The organs are preserved in University of Wisconsin solution (UW solution) and cold ischemia time is kept to a minimum (<6 hours) with good coordination between donor and recipient teams. Back table preparation may require an hour before it is ready for implantation.

Post-operative Recovery and Complications

Generally, patients need 4–6 weeks of close monitoring for recovery. Initial 2 weeks are critical because the risk of graft thrombosis, rejection and other severe complications. TPN is generally required post-operatively for a few weeks until anastomoses heal, intestinal motility and stoma output are normal. In the long term, most patients are off TPN in about a year, with few patients, especially children, requiring it for longer.

Rejection: Nearly 50% of intestine transplant recipients develop at least one episode of rejection in the first year after intestine transplantation. Acute rejection can be managed by giving a large dose of steroids or thymoglobulin. However, severe rejection is associated with substantial risk of mortality.

Infection: Sepsis due to infection, especially diarrhoea, is the most common cause of death after intestine transplantation and usually occurs along with rejection. Bacterial bloodstream and intra-abdominal infections occur in more than half of these patients. The most common viral infection is cytomegalovirus (CMV).

Renal dysfunction: These patients have a high risk for renal dysfunction compared to other organ transplants, especially because of high levels immunosuppression required in these patients to prevent rejection.

Malignancy: The most common *de novo* malignancy in these patients is due to Epstein-Barr virus (EBV) infection manifesting as post-transplant-lympho-proliferative-disorder (PTLD).

Outcomes

Intestinal transplant has become successful in the recent years. At one year, the graft-survival rates are estimated around 80% for isolated intestinal transplants and around 70% for combined liver-intestine and the multi-visceral transplant procedures with patient survival of around 90% for both. However, long-term survival rates at 10–15 years are low, about 50%. The quality of life after transplantation is better than being on TPN. Children have quality of life like normal schoolchildren.

Indian Scenario

In India, due to paucity of intestinal failure and rehabilitation services, financial constraints of long-term TPN, inability to maintain central lines for extended periods, intestinal transplantation may be appropriate early after onset of intestinal failure instead of waiting for life-threatening complications of TPN. However, a few centres offer intestinal transplant in India.

Treatment and Transplant of Pancreas

Arun Kumarraj, Somnath Chattopadhyay, Ravi Mohanka

INTRODUCTION

India has one of the highest prevalence of Type 1 Diabetes Mellitus (T1DM) in children in South Asia, i.e. 10–17 cases/1,00,000 children, in which there is auto-immune destruction of beta cells in pancreas. Pancreas transplant treats T1DM by replacing the beta cells and providing insulin. The more common type of diabetes, Type 2 (T2DM) is found in adults, its treatment by pancreas transplant is not established well.

Types

Patients requiring a pancreas transplant often also have diabetes related kidney failure and the patients with failure of both organs derive the maximum benefit from the transplant. Depending on the need for a kidney transplant, pancreas transplants are:

Simultaneous pancreas kidney (SPK) transplant: It is the most common (72%) of all pancreas transplants, performed in T1DM with end stage renal disease (ESRD), with most of these patients being on high doses to insulin and dialysis. SPK offers significant improvement in patient's lifespan as well quality of life because of freedom from insulin and dialysis.

Pancreas after kidney (PAK) transplant: It is performed in patients who has not developed ESRD, patient does not qualify for SPK listing or a living kidney donor is available. A successful pancreas transplant halts progression of ESRD and allows the patient to safely wait longer for the kidney. It comprises about 20% of all pancreas transplants.

Pancreas transplant alone (PTA): It is indicated in T1DM patients with well-preserved kidney function. PTA does not offer survival benefit compared to insulin alone, therefore, it is selectively offered to patients with life-threatening complications of DM, such as very brittle DM, multiple episodes of hyper-glycemia, hypoglycaemia unawareness and ketoacidosis. PAK comprises about 8% of pancreas transplants.

Pancreatic islet cell transplant: It involves isolation of Islet cells (insulin producing cells) from the pancreas and their transfusion into patients with DM. The cells generally get trapped in the liver and produce insulin. It is less effective in controlling DM than pancreas transplant and may require more than one session of transfusion. However, the islets are generally removed from pancreas that are not suitable for transplant as a whole organ (fatty pancreas, long cold ischemia time, etc.) and therefore it only increases access to treatment.

Donor Selection

The selection criteria for cadaveric pancreas donor is more stringent than liver or kidney donors:
- Age < 45 years
- Absence of serial increase in serum amylase levels (> 110 u/l)

- Pancreas without significant steatosis
- No history of diabetes mellitus
- BMI less than 30
- Negative tissue crossmatch (desirable)

The pancreas is prepared by attaching a Y graft on the bench before it is ready for implantation. It is therefore essential for the donor's blood vessels to be retrieved and transported with the pancreas.

Contraindications

- Severe cardiorespiratory disease
- Active infection
- Pancreatic or other malignancies
- HIV is a relative contraindication

Recipient Surgery

The pancreas is most commonly implanted in the pelvis, leaving behind the patient's own pancreas untouched with systemic venous drainage and enteric drainage of pancreatic secretions. In SPK, generally the pancreas is implanted into the right lower abdomen and the kidney in the left iliac fossa, extra-peritoneally. Other techniques such as portal venous drainage and bladder drainage for pancreatic secretions are rarely practised.

Complications

- Graft rejection
- Pancreatitis
- Vascular thrombosis
- Pancreatic exocrine leak at urinary/enteric anastomotic site

- Hypoglycemia/hyperglycemia
- Urinary disturbances
- Infection
- Bleeding

Monitoring and Postoperative Care

Patients are closely monitored for blood sugars, creatinine, proinsulin, C-Peptide, immunosuppression drug levels, apart of regular hemodynamic monitoring. In case of hyperglycmeia, a rejection may be suspected and a biopsy may be required. Generally in SPK, rejection of the kidney and pancreas happens together, therefore, a kidney biopsy (which is easier) alone may be sufficient.

Immunosuppression: Patients require standard triple drug immunosuppression, although the dose requirements may be higher than single organ alone. Patients are more prone to infection, osteoporosis, weight gain, hypertension, hyperlipidemia, nausea, vomiting.

A successful pancreas transplant not only treats T1DM, in the long term, it can reverse secondary effects of DM on other organs, such as retinopathy, neuropathy (autonomic neuropathy may take longer) and others.

Outcomes

One year pancreatic graft survival is reported at 94–96% for SPK, 85–88% for PAK and 96–99% for PTA and offers excellent survival and quality of life benefits. PTA should be offered to very selected patients. There is a large population of children suffering from T1DM who could benefit from pancreas transplant.

Heart and Lungs

Anatomy and Physiology of Heart and Lungs

Balaji Aironi

The heart is a muscular organ located between the lungs, in the middle compartment of the chest. It pumps blood through the blood vessels of the circulatory system. Blood provides oxygen and nutrients to the body, as well as removes wastes from the body.

There is a sac called pericardium, which encloses the heart, and it has a small amount of fluid inside.

In humans, the heart is divided into four chambers: Upper left and right atria and lower left and right ventricles. Commonly the right atrium and right ventricle are referred together as the right heart and their left counterpart as the left heart (Fig. 1.1).

The atrium is always smaller in size than the ventricle and they have thinner, muscle wall. They receive blood. The atria act as receiving

Anterior view

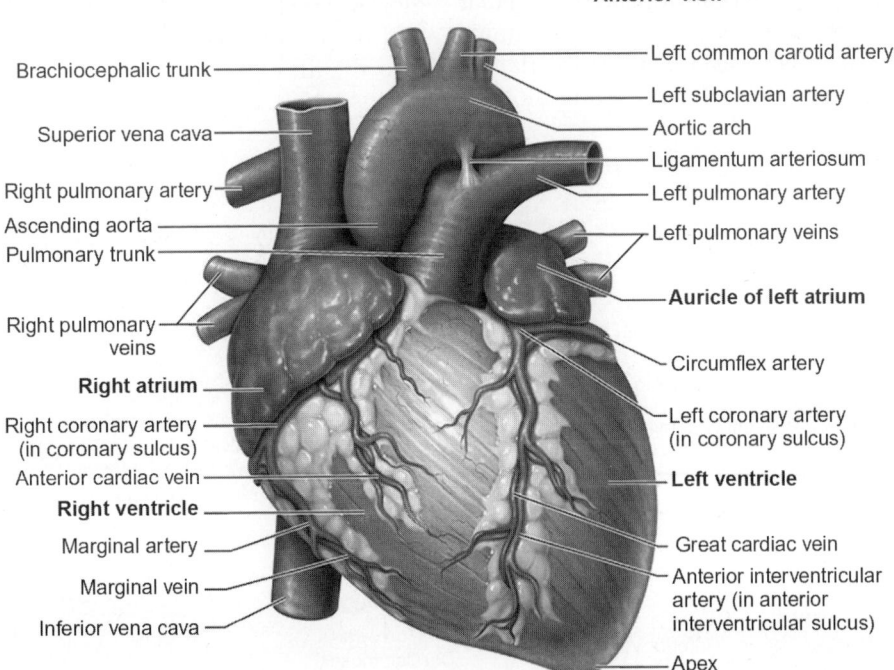

Brachiocephalic trunk

Superior vena cava

Right pulmonary artery

Ascending aorta

Pulmonary trunk

Right pulmonary veins

Right atrium

Right coronary artery (in coronary sulcus)

Anterior cardiac vein

Right ventricle

Marginal artery

Marginal vein

Inferior vena cava

Left common carotid artery

Left subclavian artery

Aortic arch

Ligamentum arteriosum

Left pulmonary artery

Left pulmonary veins

Auricle of left atrium

Circumflex artery

Left coronary artery (in coronary sulcus)

Left ventricle

Great cardiac vein

Anterior interventricular artery (in anterior interventricular sulcus)

Apex

Fig 1.1: Gross anatomy of heart

chambers for blood. The right atrium receives impure (deoxygenated) blood from SVC (superior vena cava) and IVC (inferior vena cava). SVC receives blood from upper part of the body and the IVC from the lower part of body and abdomen. The right atrium is connected to the right ventricle through tricuspid valve.

The left atrium receives (oxygenated) pure blood from lungs through the six pulmonary veins. The left atrium is connected to the left ventricle through a mitral valve.

The ventricles are the larger, stronger pumping chambers that send blood out of the heart. The right ventricle is connected to pulmonary artery with pulmonary valve within. This carries impure blood from right atrium to the lungs for purification (oxygenation).

The left ventricle is connected to aorta with an aortic valve within. The aorta carries pure oxygenated blood from the left atrium to the whole body.

The heart wall is made of 3 layers: Epicardium, myocardium and endocardium (Fig. 1.2).
- *Epicardium*: The epicardium is the outer-most layer of the heart wall that helps to lubricate and protect the outside of the heart.
- *Myocardium*: The myocardium is the muscular middle layer of the heart wall that contains the **cardiac muscle tissue** and is the part of the heart responsible for pumping blood.

- *Endocardium.* The endocardium is very smooth and prevents blood from sticking to the inside of the heart and forming potentially deadly blood clots.

Blood flows one way through the heart due to heart valves, which prevents backflow.

Heart tissue, like all cells in the body, needs oxygen and nutrients and is achieved by the coronary circulation, which includes coronary arteries and veins.

The heart pumps blood with a rhythm determined by the conduction system of heart. A pacemaker called sinoatrial node located in the right atrium determines the rate and rhythm of the heart.

Lungs

The lungs are a spongy, air-filled organ located on either side of the chest within the rib cage. The lungs form the important organ of the respiratory system and deals with the gaseous exchange from blood. This purifies the blood (i.e. removes carbon dioxide and oxygenates the blood).

The lungs are divided into the airway system and the lungs proper. The airway system consists of windpipe that originates from the glottis. Trachea then divides into the bronchi and the bronchioles. These bronchioles open into the alveoli, called the respiratory unit. This is where the gaseous exchange occurs.

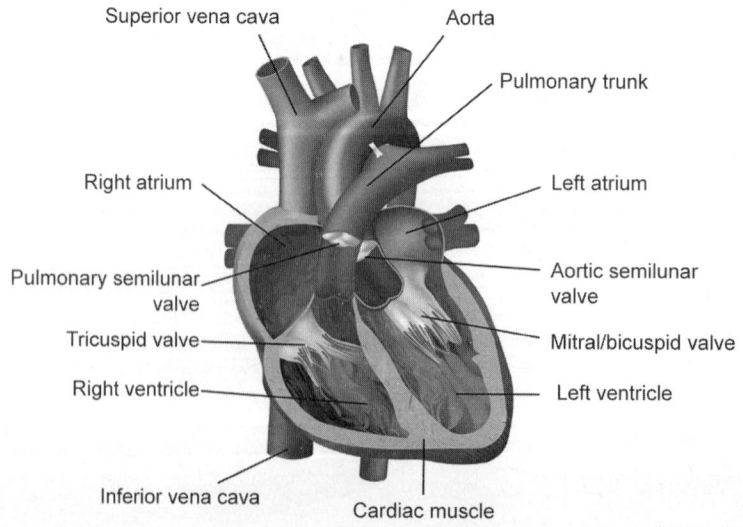

Fig 1.2: Internal anatomy of heart

The lungs are divided into the right and the left lung which in turn divides into the lobes. Lobes are further divided into the lobules and then the alveoli.

The lungs are connected to the heart through the hilum of lungs containing pulmonary artery and the pulmonary veins (Fig. 1.3).

Physiology of Gas Exchange

The pulmonary artery gets impure blood from the heart (right ventricle) to the lungs. And at the alveolar level the blood gets purified, i.e. the carbon dioxide is removed and oxygen is added to the blood. The exchange of gases takes place due to pressure difference of the gases in blood and the air that is inspired (breathe in). This process of gas exchange is called diffusion. The purified blood is then drained by the pulmonary veins that connect to the left atrium of the heart (Fig. 1.4).

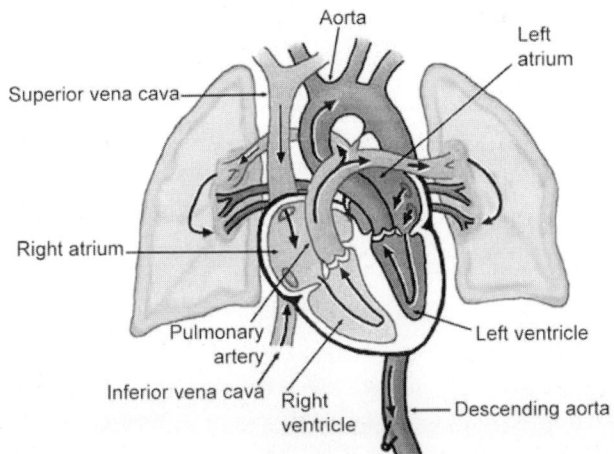

Fig. 1.3: Cardiopulmonary circulation

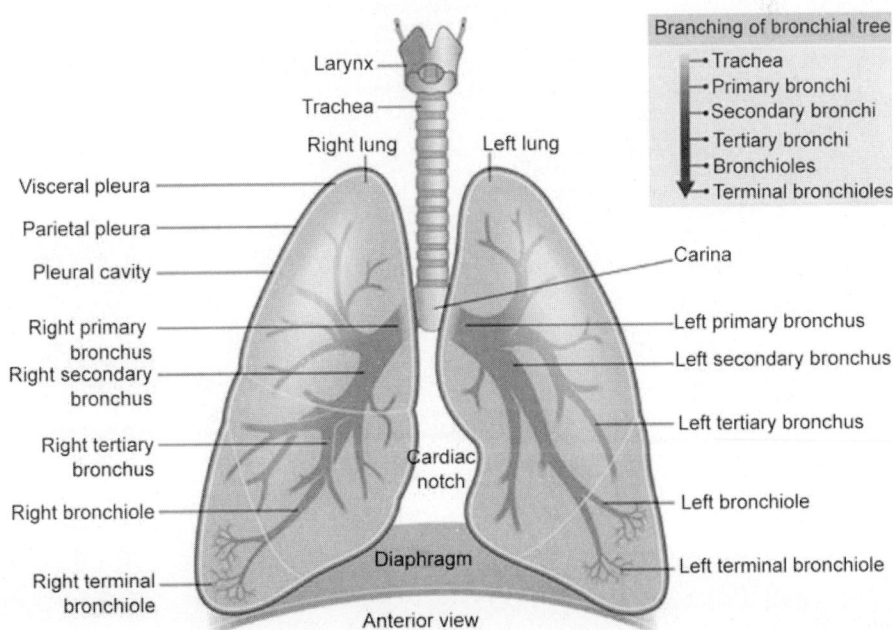

Fig. 1.4: Gross anatomy of the lungs

Indications for Heart Transplantation

Heart transplantation is done for patients with end-stage congestive heart failure (CHF) who will not live for more than 1 year without intervention, transplant and who are not candidates for or have not been helped by conventional medical therapy. Specific indications for a transplant include the following:

- Dilated cardiomyopathy
- Ischemic cardiomyopathy
- Congenital heart disease for which no conventional therapy exists or for which conventional therapy has failed
- Ejection fraction of less than 20%
- Intractable angina or malignant cardiac arrhythmias for which conventional therapy has been exhausted
- Age younger than 65 years
- Ability to comply with medical follow-up care

Indications for Lung Transplant

Lung transplants are indicated for patients with end-stage lung disease for which maximal medical therapy is ineffective or there is no proven therapy. These include patients with the following diseases or conditions:

- Idiopathic pulmonary fibrosis (IPF)
- Chronic obstructive pulmonary disease (COPD)
- Cystic fibrosis
- Idiopathic pulmonary arterial hypertension
- Sarcoidosis
- Lymphangioleyomyomatosis (LAM).

Prevention of Heart Disease

Bharat Shivdasani, Saurabh Dhariya

INTRODUCTION

Cardiovascular disease (CVD) continues to be the leading cause of death in the United States and other developed countries. The burden from CVD has been increasing in developing countries as well. According to current projections, overall CVD rates will continue to increase in the twenty-first century and will be the leading cause of death in both developed and the developing nations. The large global burden of CVD is occurring despite the availability of proven primary and secondary preventive strategies that have not been effectively disseminated. However, before a large-scale CVD prevention program is implemented, key decision-makers must be aware of the scope of the problem.

Coronary heart disease is characterised by insufficient circulation in coronary arteries potentially leading to angina pectoris (chest pain), heart failure and sudden coronary death. Underlying pathophysiology is most often coronary atherosclerosis and is largely preventable by controlling the common risk factors.

Epidemiology

With the turn of the century, cardiovascular diseases (CVDs) have become the leading cause of mortality in India. In comparison with the people of European ancestry, CVD affects Indians at least a decade earlier and in their most productive midlife years.

In addition, case fatality attributable to CVD in low-income countries, including India, appears to be much higher than in middle- and high-income countries. The World Health Organization (WHO) has estimated that with the current burden of CVD, India would lose $237 billion from the loss of productivity and spending on health care over a 10-year period (2005–2015).

The epidemiological transition in India in the past 2 decades has been dramatic; in a short timeframe, the predominant epidemiological characteristics have transitioned from infectious diseases, diseases of undernutrition, and maternal and childhood diseases to noncommunicable diseases (NCDs).

CVD is the leading cause of death in all parts of India, including the poorer states and rural areas.

According to the Global Burden of Disease study age-standardized estimates (2010), nearly a quarter (24.8%) of all deaths in India are attributable to CVD (Fig. 2.1).

Risk factors for cardiovascular disease: Can be divided into:

Modifiable	Non-modifiable
Tobacco smoking	Age
High blood cholesterol and triglyceride	Gender
Physical inactivity	Family history
Obesity or overweight	
Diet	
Individual response to stress	

Psychosocial index
High blood pressure
Alcohol consumption
Diabetes
Metabolic syndrome

Individual Risk Factor Stratification and Prevention

Smoking

Other than advanced age, smoking remains the single most important risk factor for

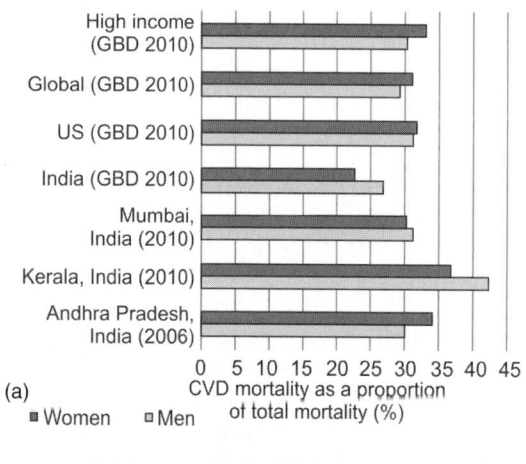

(a)

■ Women   ▫ Men

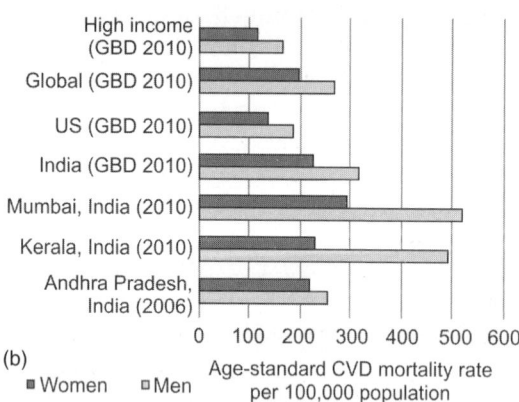

(b)

■ Women   ▫ Men

Fig. 2.1: a. Proportion of cardiovascular diseases mortailty in India based on data from available prospective studies and global burden of disease estimates.[11] The prospective studies included in the figure and Pednekar, et. al.[13] Soman, et. al.[14] (Kerala, Urban and Rural), and Joshi, et. al.[15] (Andhra Pradesh, Rural); b. Age-standardized rate of cardiovascular disease mortality in India based on Global Burden of disease estimates and data from available prospective studies.[11] CVD indicates cardiovascular disease; and GBD (global burden of disease)

coronary artery disease. Smokers lose at least one decade of life expectancy, as compared with never-smokers.

The risk of death from cigarette smoking continues to increase among women and the increased risks are now nearly identical for men and women. Compared with nonsmokers, smoking increases the risk of both coronary heart disease and stroke two- to fourfold. Ischemic heart disease underlies 35% to 40% of all smoking-related deaths, with an additional 8% attributable to second hand smoke exposure. Cigarette smoking can promote vasoconstriction, resulting in a greater risk of developing symptomatic peripheral vascular disease and abdominal aortic aneurysm among smokers than nonsmokers. Second hand smoke exposure is also associated with heart disease in non-smoking adults.

Passive smoking , either at home or work, is known to increase the risk of heart disease by 25 to 30%

"Light" levels of smoking have a major impact on MI and all-cause mortality. Continued smoking is also a major risk factor for recurrent MI.

Beyond acute unfavorable effects on blood pressure and sympathetic tone and a reduction in myocardial oxygen supply, smoking contributes to the pathogenesis of athero-thrombosis by several other mechanisms. Long-term smoking may enhance oxidation of LDL cholesterol and impair endothelium-dependent coronary artery vasodilation. This latter effect has been linked to dysfunctional endothelial nitric oxide biosynthesis with chronic as well as acute cigarette consumption. In addition, smoking has adverse hemostatic and inflammatory effects, including increases in levels of C-reactive protein (CRP), soluble intercellular adhesion molecule-1 (ICAM-1), fibrinogen, and homocysteine. Additionally, smoking is associated with spontaneous platelet aggregation, increased monocyte adhesion to endothelial cells, and adverse alterations in endothelium-derived fibrinolytic and anti-thrombotic factors, including tissue-type plasminogen activator and tissue pathway factor inhibitor. Compared with nonsmokers,

smokers have an increased prevalence of coronary spasm and a reduced threshold for ventricular arrhythmias. Accruing evidence has suggested that insulin resistance represents an additional mechanistic link between smoking and premature atherosclerosis.

Interventions for Smoking Cessation

Smoking cessation is by far the major preventive intervention to reduce cardiovascular mortality. This cessation of smoking benefits risk reductions equal or exceed those for other secondary prevention interventions that have received more attention from physicians and the pharmaceutical industry, including the use of aspirin, statins, beta-adrenergic blocking agents, and angiotensin-converting enzyme (ACE) inhibitors. Smoking cessation approaches include brief clinical interventions (e.g. a physician taking 10 minutes or less to deliver advice and assistance about quitting); counseling (e.g. individual, group, or telephone counseling); behavioral cessation therapies (e.g. training in problem solving); and treatments with more person-to-person contact and intensity. Cessation medications found to be effective for treating tobacco dependence include nicotine replacement products, either over-the-counter (e.g. nicotine patch, gum, lozenge) or prescription (e.g. nicotine inhaler, nasal spray), and prescription non-nicotine medications such as bupropion SR, varenicline tartrate, or new agents such as cytisine. Preventing smoking in the first place should receive greater emphasis. Community education and physician-based primary prevention remain the most important components of any smoking reduction strategy.

Hypertension

Elevated blood pressure is a major risk factor for coronary heart disease, heart failure, cerebrovascular disease, peripheral arterial disease, renal failure, atrial fibrillation, and total mortality, as well as loss of cognitive function and dementia. Though the degree of blood pressure lowering relates linearly to risk reduction, it should not be treated alone, but include assessment of all cardiovascular risk factors in a holistic approach, incorporating patient-centered lifestyle modification. Prehypertension, defined as systolic blood pressure between 120 and 139 mm Hg or diastolic blood pressure between 80 and 89 mm Hg, is associated with nearly twice the risk of MI and stroke in women compared with normal blood pressure. Hypertension often confers silent cardiovascular risk. High blood pressure is defined as systolic blood pressure of 140 mm Hg or greater or diastolic blood pressure of 90 mm Hg or greater or taking antihypertensive medicine.

Ambulatory monitoring of blood pressure over 24 hours may provide a stronger predictor of cardiovascular morbidity and mortality than office-based measures.

Prevention and Management of Hypertension

Diet and lifestyle management remain the cornerstone of prevention of hypertension, and clinical trial evidence continues to accrue showing that adopting low-risk dietary measures along with weight reduction, particularly at the societal level, could substantially reduce the burden of blood pressure. Routine pharmacologic therapy for prehypertension in the presence of other major comorbid conditions such as diabetes, renal dysfunction, or known vascular disease should await further evidence of benefit. For all patients with blood pressure of 120/80 mm Hg or greater, lifestyle modifications including smoking cessation, weight reduction if needed, increased physical activity, limited alcohol intake, limited sodium intake, adequate potassium and calcium intake, and adoption of the Dietary Approaches to Stop Hypertension (DASH) eating plan, a diet with a reduced content of saturated and total fat that also includes abundant fruits, vegetables, and low-fat dairy products. Initiation of drug therapy depends on blood pressure and the absolute level of risk. Most patients require more than one agent to achieve their blood pressure goals.

Metabolic Syndrome, Insulin Resistance and Diabetes Mellitus

Insulin resistance and diabetes rank among the major cardiovascular risk factors; the presence of diabetes confers an equivalent risk to aging 15 years, an impact comparable with if not greater than that of smoking. Compared with unaffected persons, diabetic patients have a greater atherosclerotic burden in the major arteries, as well as of microvascular disease. Not surprisingly, diabetic patients have substantially increased rates of atherosclerotic complications in the settings of primary prevention and after coronary interventional procedures.

Moreover, the risk of cardiovascular disease starts to increase long before the onset of clinical diabetes. In an analysis of data from the Nurses Health Study on women who eventually developed type 2 diabetes, the relative risk of MI was elevated threefold before the diagnosis of diabetes, for a cardiovascular event rate almost as high as the rate in patients with Frank diabetes at study entry. Although several formal definitions of the metabolic syndrome have been proposed, the definition adopted by the National Cholesterol Education Program Adult Treatment Panel requires at least three of the following five criteria: (1) waist circumference larger than 102 cm in men and 88 cm in women; (2) serum triglyceride levels of at least 150 mg/dl; (3) HDL cholesterol less than 40 mg/dl in men and less than 50 mg/dl in women; (4) blood pressure of at least 130/85 mm Hg; and (5) serum glucose concentration of at least 110 mg/dl.

In addition to systemic metabolic abnormalities, hyperglycemia causes accumulation of advanced glycation end products associated with vascular damage. Diabetic patients have impaired endothelial vasodilator function and appear to have increased leukocyte adhesion to vascular endothelium, a critical early step in atherogenesis. Diabetic nephropathy, detected by microalbuminuria, accelerates these adverse processes. Among persons with non-insulin-dependent diabetes, microalbuminuria predicts cardiovascular and all-cause mortality.

Interventions to Reduce Cardiovascular Risk Among Diabetic Patients

Whether pre-diabetes *per se* produces atherosclerosis and its complications is uncertain. Pre-diabetes is known to be associated with metabolic syndrome which is a known risk factor for macrovascular disease. It also worsens with age, thereby justifying intervention for CVD risk factors in all such patients. First-line management is lifestyle intervention: Weight reduction in obese subjects, reduced intakes of dietary saturated and trans-fatty acids, cholesterol, and sodium, and increased physical activity. The use of drugs to control CVD risk factors likewise deserves consideration.

Targets of therapy include dyslipidemia, hypertension, and prothrombotic factors. Dyslipidemic parameters that need control are lower density lipoproteins (LDL) and very LDL which are known to be atherogenic. In patients with CVD plus metabolic syndrome, LDL cholesterol levels should be reduced to <70 mg/dl, and LDL + very LDL cholesterol (non-HDL cholesterol) to <100 mg/dl.[20] Statins are first-line drugs to achieve these reductions. If these goals are not attained with a statin, a second-line LDL-lowering drug can be used: Nicotinic acid, bile acid sequestrant, or ezetimibe. If CVD is not present, goals are an LDL cholesterol <100 mg/dl and a non-HDL cholesterol <130 mg/dl. In most patients, a statin alone usually is sufficient to achieve this goal.

Blood pressure should be lowered to <130/<85 mm Hg, and preferably to <120/<80 mm Hg. Any of the standard blood pressure lowering drugs (e.g. angiotensin-converting enzyme inhibitors/angiotensin receptor blockers, calcium blockers, diuretics, beta-blockers) can be employed. Evidence favoring 1 drug over another is limited. Nonetheless, physicians should keep in mind that beta-blockers and higher doses of thiazide diuretics raise glucose levels and predispose patients to conversion to diabetes.

Obesity

Body Mass Index (BMI) is a poor predictor of mortality risk. A combination of waist circumference or waist-hip ratio as a marker for adiposity and middle arm muscle circumference as a marker for muscle mass is a far better predictor of mortality. The mortality risk also rises in severe obesity: BMI 35 kg/sq.m in men or BMI 33 kg/sq.m in women.

Obesity is a common condition associated with increased risk for CAD and cardiovascular mortality. Excess body weight is an important factor leading to hypertension dyslipidemia, and type 2 diabetes mellitus.

A number of evidence-based recommendations have been published in the last three years, summarizing the foods, nutrients, and dietary patterns for reduction of cardiovascular disease.

Sedentary Lifestyle

Physical inactivity has been recognized as an important risk factor for CVD and HF. Prospective epidemiological studies of occupational and leisure-time physical activity have documented a reduced incidence of CAD, HF, and stroke in the more physically active and fit individuals. Increased physical activity, even by the modest amount of 30 minutes at least 5 days per week, has been documented to reduce risk for cardiovascular events. Increased physical activity has also been demonstrated to reduce the incidence of diabetes. However, the integration of physical activity into the daily lives of the population has proved challenging, and improvements will require concerted, ongoing efforts.

Several plausible biologic mechanisms can explain the cardioprotective effect of physical activity. Regular physical activity has been shown to reduce myocardial oxygen demand and increase exercise capacity (i.e. improving cardiorespiratory fitness), which correlate with lower levels of coronary risk. Physical activity also lowers systolic and diastolic blood pressure; improves insulin sensitivity and glycemic control, with major benefits for diabetic patients, including reductions in glycated hemoglobin along with reduced requirements for therapy; and improves dyslipidemia, as well as vascular inflammation. Regular physical activity is associated with lower CRP levels (particularly when adiposity decreases) and hemostatic variables including tissue-type plasminogen activator, fibrinogen, von Willebrand factor, fibrin D-dimer, and plasma viscosity. It also enhances endogenous fibrinolysis and coronary endothelial function. Physical activity helps control body weight, and lower levels of adiposity improve many of the aforementioned physiologic parameters, which are cardiovascular risk factors.

Interventions to Increase Physical Activity

A wide range of interventions were reported, with most including the use of written materials and two or more sessions of physical activity counseling, delivered face to face or by telephone. A range of professionals—including primary care physicians, nurses, physiotherapists, exercise or physical activity specialists, health educators, health promotion specialists, or trained facilitators from a range of health professions—delivered the interventions.

Diet

A large body of evidence, both from epidemiologic and intervention studies, has demonstrated that dietary factors have an important impact on coronary heart disease risk. Patterns such as the Healthy Eating Index, western versus prudent dietary patterns, Mediterranean dietary pattern, and the DASH-type diet are consistent in emphasizing fruits, vegetables, other plant foods such as beans and nuts, and in many patterns, whole grains and fish; with limited or occasional dairy products; and limiting red meats or processed meats and fewer refined carbohydrates and other processed foods. These dietary patterns conform with the food-based priorities for cardiovascular health that include foods that are higher in dietary fiber, healthy fatty acids, vitamins, antioxidants, potassium, other minerals, and phytochemicals, and lower in refined carbohydrates, sugars, salt, saturated fatty acids, dietary cholesterol, and trans fat.

Alcohol Consumption

Habitual heavy alcohol consumption increases total mortality, cardiovascular disease mortality, coronary heart disease, and stroke. By contrast, a consistent body of observational epidemiologic evidence has shown that light to moderate alcohol consumption, compared with nondrinkers, associates inversely with risk of heart attack, ischemic stroke, peripheral vascular disease, sudden cardiac death, diabetes mellitus, and death from all cardiovascular causes.

Any individual or public health recommendation must consider the complexity of alcohol's metabolic, physiologic, and psychological effects. The 2010 Dietary Guidelines for Americans recommend that if alcohol is consumed, it should be consumed in moderation—up to one drink (30 ml) per day for women and two drinks per day for men—and only by adults of legal drinking age. With alcohol, the difference between daily intake of small to moderate quantities and large quantities may tip the balance between preventing and causing disease. Because of the health hazards of alcohol associated with higher intake, moderate alcohol use does not offer a desirable population based strategy to reduce cardiovascular risk

Conclusion

Control of modifiable risk factors will result in significant reduction in the occurrence of ischemic heart disease. Primary prevention in the society will play a great role in reducing the burden of heart disease.

Further Reading

1. Chobanian AV, Bakris GL, Black HR, et al: Seventh report of the Joint National Committee on Pre-vention, Detection, Evaluation, and Treatment of High Blood Pressure. Hypertension 42:1206, 2003. 2.

2. Cook NR, Paynter NP, Eaton CB, et al: Com-parison of the Framingham and Reynolds risk scores for global cardiovascular risk prediction in the multiethnic Women's Health Initiative. Circulation 125:1748, 2012.

3. Dorairaj Prabhakaran, et al. Cardiovascular Diseases in India Current Epidemiology and Future Directions; Circulation. 2016;133:1605–1620. DOI: 10.1161/CIRCULATIONAHA.114.008729.

4. Ebrahim S, Taylor F, Ward K, Beswick A, Burke M, Davey Smith G. Multiple risk factor int erventions for primary prevention of coronary heart disease. Cochrane Database Syst Rev2011;1: CD001561.

5. Go AS, Mozaffarian D, Roger VL, et al: Heart disease and stroke statistics—2013 update: A report from the American Heart Association. Circulation 127:e6, 2013.

6. Gregory L. Burke and Ronny A. Bell: National and International Trends in Cardiovascular Disease: Incidence and Risk Factors. preventive cardiology A companion to Braunwalds heart disease; page 14.

7. Hu FB, Stampfer MJ, Haffner SM, et al: Elevated risk of cardiovascular disease prior to clinical diagnosis of type 2 diabetes. Diabetes Care 25: 1129, 2002.

8. Institute of Health Metrics and Evaluation. GBD Profile: India. http://WWW.healthdata.org / sites/default/files/files/country_profiles/ GBD/ihme_gbd_country_report_india.pdf. accessedapril 30, 2014.

9. Institute of Health Metrics and Evaluation: GBD Compare2010 .http:// vizhub. Healthdata. org / gbd-compare/. Accessed April 30, 2014.

10. Jha P, Ramasundarahettige C, Landsman V, et al: 21st-century hazards of smoking and benefits of cessation in the United States. N Engl J Med 368:341, 2013.

11. Joshi P, Islam S, Pais P, Reddy S, Dorairaj P, Kazmi K, Pandey MR, Haque S, Mendis S, Rangarajan S, Yusuf S. Risk factors for early myocardial infarction in South Asians compared with individuals in other countries. JAMA. 2007; 297:286–294. doi: 10.1001/jama.297.3.286.

12. Katsunori Nonogaki Dysglycemia and Cardio-vascular Risk Journal of the American College of Cardiology, Volume 60, Issue 12, 18 September 2012, Pages 1121.

13. Lichtman JH, Bigger JT, Jr, Blumenthal JA, et al: Depression and coronary heart disease: Recommendations for screening, referral, and treatment: A science advisory from the American Heart Association Prevention Committee of the Council On Cardiovascular Nursing, Council on Clinical Cardiology, Council on Epidemiology and Prevention, and Interdisciplinary Council on Quality of Care and Outcomes Research: Endorsed by the American Psychiatric Association. Circulation 118:1768, 2008.

14. Moran AE, Forouzanfar MH, Roth GA, Mensah GA, Ezzati M, Murray CJ,Naghavi M. Temporal

trends in ischemic heart disease mortality in 21 world regions, 1980 to 2010: the Global Burden of Disease 2010 study. Circulation2014;129:1483–1492.

15. Mozaffarian D, Appel LJ, Van Horn L: Components of a cardioprotective diet: New insights. Circulation 123:2870, 2011.

16. Prabhakaran D, Yusuf S, Mehta S, Pogue J, Avezum A, Budaj A, Cerumzynski L, Flather M, Fox K, Hunt D, Lisheng L, Keltai M, Parkhomenko A, Pais P, Reddy S, Ruda M, Hiquing T, Jun Z. Two-year outcomes in patients admitted with non-ST elevation acute coronary syndrome: results of the OASIS registry 1 and 2. Indian Heart J. 2005; 57:217–22.

17. Report on Causes of Death in India 2001–2003. New Delhi, India: Office of the Registrar General of India; 2009.

18. Si S, Moss JR, Sullivan TR, Newton SS, Stocks NP. Effectiveness of general practice-based health checks: a systematic review and meta-analysis.Br J Gen Pract2014;64:e47–e53.

19. Srinath Reddy K, Shah B, Varghese C, Ramadoss A. Responding to the threat of chronic diseases in India. Lancet. 2005;366:1744–1749. doi: 10.1016/ S0140-6736(05)67343–6.

20. Thun MJ, Carter BD, Feskanich D, et al: 50-year trends in smoking-related mortality in the United States. N Engl J Med 368:351, 2013.

21. US. Department of Health and Human Services: 2008 physical activity guidelines for Americans. 2008. (http://www.health.gov/paguidelines/ pdf/paguide).

22. Wang L, McLeod HL, Weinshilboum RM: Genomics and drug response. N Engl J Med 364:1144, 2011.

23. Xavier D, Pais P, Devereaux PJ, Xie C, Prabhakaran D, Reddy KS, Gupta R, Joshi P, Kerkar P, Thanikachalam S, Haridas KK, Jaison TM, Naik S, Maity AK, Yusuf S; CREATE registry investigators. Treatment and outcomes of acute coronary syndromes in India (CREATE): a prospective analysis of registry data. Lancet. 2008;371:1435–1442. doi: 10.1016/ S0140-6736(08) 60623–6.

24. Yusuf S, Rangarajan S, Teo K, Islam S, Li W, Liu L, Bo J, Lou Q, Lu F, Liu T, Yu L, Zhang S, Mony P, Swaminathan S, Mohan V, Gupta R, Kumar R, Vijayakumar K, Lear S, Anand S, Wielgosz A, Diaz R, Avezum A, LopezJaramillo P, Lanas F, Yusoff K, Ismail N, Iqbal R, Rahman O, Rosengren A, Yusufali A, Kelishadi R, Kruger A, Puoane T, Szuba A, Chifamba J, Oguz A, McQueen M, McKee M, Dagenais G; PURE Investigators. Cardiovascular risk and events in 17 low-, middle-, and high-income countries. N Engl J Med. 2014; 371:818–827. doi: 10.1056/NEJMoa1311890.

Prevention of Lung Diseases and Overview of Lung Transplantation

SP Rai

The Lungs: An Overview of how they Work

Every part of your body needs oxygen from the air you breathe in order to survive. The lungs are designed to absorb oxygen from the air and transfer it to the bloodstream.

The lungs are found inside the chest and are protected by the rib cage. Between the ribs are muscles that are essential for breathing. The most important muscle of breathing is called the diaphragm. It is dome-shaped and lies below the lungs separating them from the abdomen. The lungs are made up of several conducting airways, the smallest of which end in tiny air sacs called alveoli. These air sacs have very thin walls which are criss-crossed with hundreds of tiny blood vessels called capillaries. There are 200 million or so of these air sacs (Fig. 3.1).

What Makes you Breathe?

The breathing center in the brain is constantly receiving signals from the body about the amount of oxygen which is needed. This will depend on how active you are. Breathing occurs when the breathing centre in the brain sends a message along the nerves to your

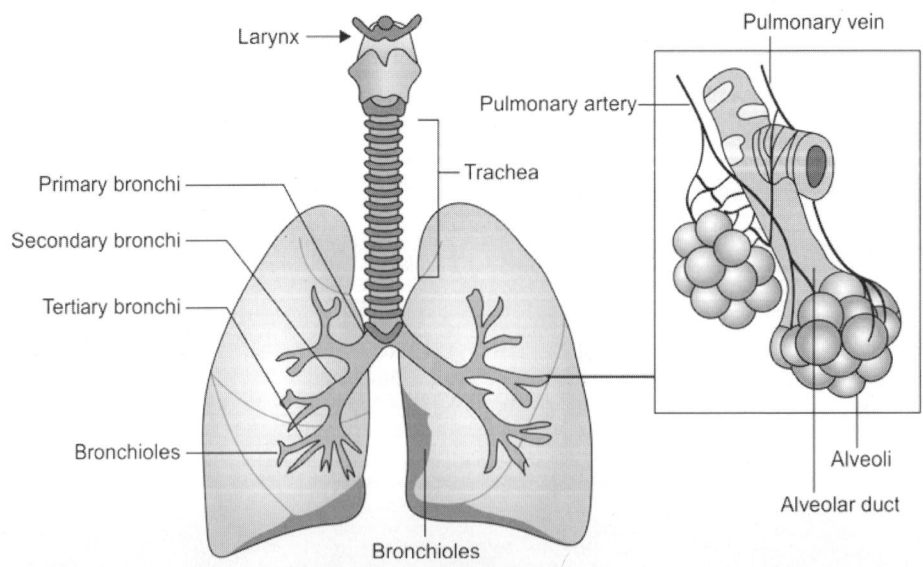

Fig. 3.1: Basic anatomy of the lungs

breathing muscles. The muscles contract and you breathe in. Each time you breathe, air is drawn into your lungs through your airways. The air passes down the bronchi which divide another 15 to 25 times into thousands of smaller and smaller airways, called bronchioles, until the air reaches the alveoli. Breathing out is due to the elastic recoil of the lungs so that the air is pushed out and the lungs return to their resting size.

How does Oxygen Get into the Bloodstream?

Inside the alveoli, oxygen moves across the paper thin walls of the capillaries, and into the blood, where it is picked up by hemoglobin in the red blood cells ready to be carried around the body. At the same time, a by-product from metabolism of cells, tissues in the body called carbon dioxide, comes out of the capillaries back into the alveoli, ready to be breathed out (Fig. 3.2). Freshly oxygenated blood is carried from the lungs to the heart which pumps blood around the body through the arteries. Once the oxygen has been used up in the tissues of the body, the blood returns, through the veins, to the heart. It is then pumped to the lungs so that the carbon dioxide can be removed and more oxygen taken up.

What Else do Lungs do?

With about 10,000 liters of air moving in and out of the lungs every day, germs and other foreign bodies can also find their way into the airways. The lungs are provided with a number of complex defense systems to prevent unwanted material from getting into the body. Mucus produced in the walls of the airways helps to trap any particles. Antibodies are produced which protect against foreign and unwanted inhaled material and germs. Tiny hairs line the bronchi and help move unwanted materials up to the mouth where they can be coughed out or blown into a handkerchief or tissue. The delicate structure of the lungs is beautifully adapted to carry out the complex business of breathing and, at the same time, helps protect the body from outside attack. Most of the time we are not even aware that our lungs are working, but they can be damaged in many ways and become less efficient at taking oxygen from the air and getting rid of waste carbon dioxide.

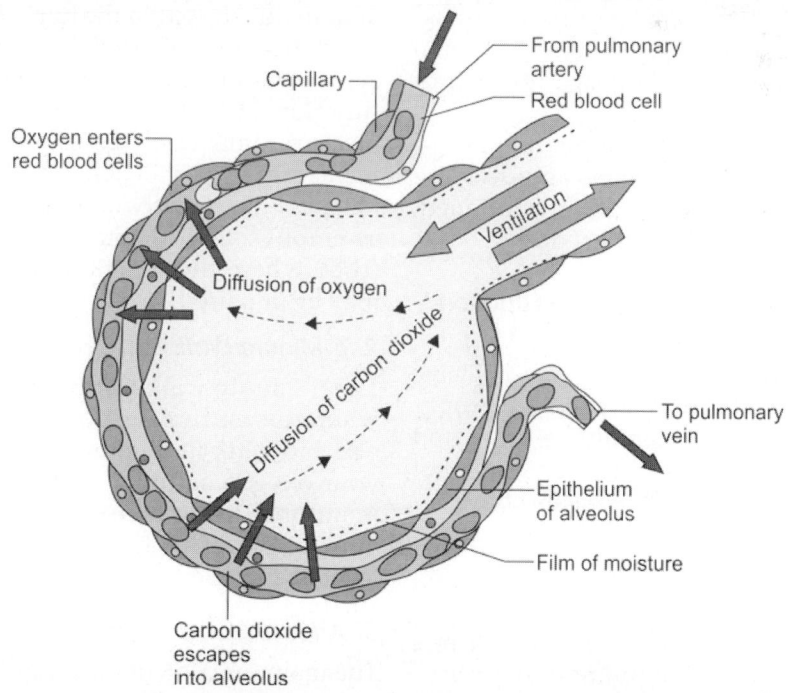

Fig. 3.2: Structure of the alveolus

Everyday we breathe about 22,000 times. It is important to pay attention to the health of lung as the basic function of breathing is often neglected. As the symptom of lung disease come on very slowly, the patient may not seek early medical care.

Check in with Your Lungs

If You

- Have a new, persistent or changed cough?
- Cough up mucus, phlegm or blood?
- Get breathless more easily than others your age?
- Experience chest tightness or wheeze?
- Have frequent chest infections?
- Experience chest pain, fatigue or sudden weight loss?

If you have any of these, your lung health could be at risk... particularly if you

- Smoke or have ever smoked?
- Work or worked in a job that exposed you to dust, gas or fumes?

Consult your doctor, if you experience these symptoms.

Lung Function Tests

Lung function tests measure the functional capacity of the lungs and are important investigations which:
- Help diagnose suspected lung disease
- Help in planning treatments and deciding whether treatments should be continued, changed, or are no longer needed

How does it Feel to Perform Lung Function Tests?

Lung function tests are mostly non-invasive but require good efforts to produce proper results. This may occasionally be tiring and make you feel a bit puffed, but is usually not uncomfortable and only lasts a short time.

Types of Lung Function Tests

1. Spirometry (Fig. 3.3)

Common lung conditions, such as asthma and chronic obstructive pulmonary disease (COPD), cause problems by narrowing the

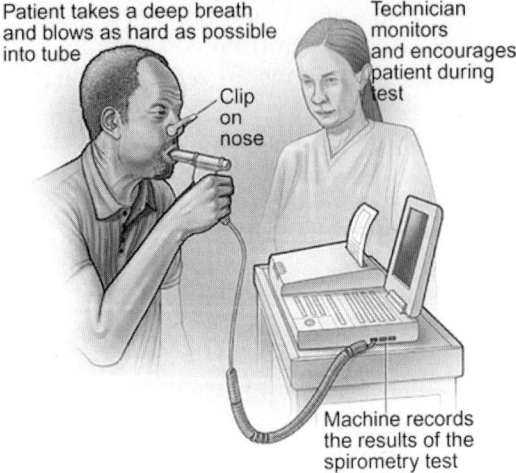

Patient takes a deep breath and blows as hard as possible into tube

Clip on nose

Technician monitors and encourages patient during test

Machine records the results of the spirometry test

Fig. 3.3: Performing a spirometry

airways (bronchial tubes) resulting in shortness of breath. Spirometry is a simple test to measure the narrowing in the respiratory track. At value for measuring exactly how much narrowing is present. Measurements such as the forced expiratory volume in 1 second (FEV1) and forced vital capacity (FVC) are made, which indicate the presence, site and severity of airway narrowing (FEV1) and the quantity of air within the lungs (FVC).

The transport of oxygen and corbon dioxide across the alveolar membrane is the basic function of the lung. A gas diffusion test measures how easily gases pass through this membrane. This valuable information is used to assess the severity of lung conditions such as emphysema and interstitial lung disease (ILD) where the function of the membrane may be impaired.

2. 6-Minute Walk Test

The 6-minute walk test is a very simple test where measurements are made of how far you can walk in 6 minutes. During the test, your oxygen saturations and heart rate are monitored using an oximeter on the end of your finger. This helps to determine your level of exercise capacity.

3. Arterial Blood Gases

The main function of the lungs is to transport oxygen into the bloodstream and remove waste carbon dioxide from the blood. An arterial sample of the blood is used to measure the amount of oxygen and carbon dioxide in the blood. In patients with compressed lung function, the oxygen value is less and carbon dioxide value is more.

Prevent Lung Disease

Take good care of your lungs, and they can last you a lifetime. Treat them poorly and you run the risk of developing lung disease. There are more than 30 different types of lung diseases ranging from tuberculosis, asthma, cystic fibrosis and chronic obstructive pulmonary disease to lung cancer and pneumonia. Below are some tips to keep your lungs healthy.

1. Don't smoke... Anything

Smoking is dangerous and causes lung cancer and COPD. Smoking releases harmful substances in the lung and hence one should not smoke. If you are still smoking, it is never too late to quit. Also, make sure kids understand the dangers of smoking and be a role model by not smoking or by committing to quit. Do not allow smoking in your home, in the car, or at work. The tobacco fumes stick to the walls, furniture, carpet in the house and are damaging to the lung. Paint the walls with low valatile organic compounds (VOC) paints.

2. Prevent Infection

A cold or other respiratory infection can sometimes become very serious. There are several ways to protect yourself:
- Wash your hands often with soap and water. Alcohol-based cleaners are a good substitute if you cannot wash.
- Avoid crowds during the cold and flu season.
- Cover you coughs. To help stop the spread of germs, cover your mouth and nose with a tissue when you cough or sneeze. Wear a face mask.
- Good oral hygiene can protect you from the germs in your mouth leading to infections. Brush your teeth at least twice daily.
- Get vaccinated every year against influenza and ask your health care provider about pneumococcal vaccinations.

- If you get sick, keep a distance from others by approximately 6 feet. Stay home from work or school until you're feeling better.

Asthma and COPD must be kept under regular treatment from the doctor. Preventive medications, such as inhaled corticosteroids, can cut your risk of asthma attacks, and rescue medications, such as salbutamol inhalers, can stop symptoms like coughing or wheezing. Know your triggers, and avoid them, if possible. Also do your best to avoid respiratory infections, which can exacerbate both the conditions.

3. Clean House

Air fresheners, mould, pet dander, dust mites and construction materials all pose a potential problem. Turn on the exhaust fan when you cook and avoid using aerosol products like hair spray.

4. Check your Home for Radon

Radon gas (a naturally occurring radioactive gas produced by the breakdown of uranium in the ground) is a hidden killer and the second leading cause of lung cancer after smoking. Find out if there are high levels of radon in your home or workplace. It may be leaking into the house through cracks in the foundation and walls.

5. Wear a Mask

Workers may be exposed to an excessive amount of dust, fumes, smoke, gases, vapors or mists in the workplace. Poor ventilation, closed-in working areas and heat increase are also disease-causing culprits. Avoid breathing in toxic fumes from chemical, solvents and paints. Wear protective masks when you work with chemicals and report unsafe working conditions. Go to lung screening and other health programs offered at work.

6. Stay Active

Lungs at rest and during most daily activities are only 50% of their capacity. To help counteract the build-up of toxins and tar in the lung caused by environmental pollutants, allergens, dust and cigarette smoke, you need to help your lungs cleanse themselves. Regular modestly intense activity is great for the lungs. Aim for at least 20 minutes of consistent, moderately intense movement daily, like a brisk walk or a bike ride.

Diaphragmatic breathing

Diaphragmatic breathing uses the awareness of the diaphragm muscle, which separates the organs in the abdomen from your lungs. By concentrating on lowering the diaphragm as you breathe in, you will get a much deeper inhale.

Simple deep breathing

Deep breathing can get you closer to reaching your lungs' full capacity. As you inhale, consciously expand your belly with awareness of lowering the diaphragm. Next expand your ribs, allowing the floating ribs to open like wings. Finally, allow the upper chest to expand and lift. After this, exhale as completely as possible by letting the chest fall, then contracting the ribs and, finally, bring the stomach muscles in and up to lift the diaphragm and expel the last bit of air.

Counting on your breath

You can also increase your lung capacity by increasing the length of your inhalations and exhalations. Start by counting how long a natural breath takes. If it takes to count to five to inhale it should take the count to five to exhale. You will want them to be of equal length. Once you have discovered the count of your average breath, add one more count to each inhale and exhale until you can comfortably extend the length of time it takes to fill and empty your lungs. The point is to avoid straining or being uncomfortable. It should be a gradual and easy process.

Making room: Watch your posture

Since your lungs are soft structures, they only take up the room that you make for them. A simple technique for giving your lungs more room is leaning back slightly in a stable chair, lifting the chest and opening the front of your body as you breathe deeply.

7. Incentive Spirometry

Postoperative pulmonary complications are reported in the range of 2–39% and include atelectasis, pneumonia, and respiratory failure. Upper abdominal surgical procedures are associated with a higher risk of complications, followed by lower abdominal surgery and thoracic surgery. Preoperative and postoperative respiratory therapy aims to prevent or reverse atelectasis and improve airway clearance. The risk and severity of complications can be reduced by the use of therapeutic maneuvers that increase lung volume. Incentive spirometry has been routinely considered a part of the perioperative respiratory therapy strategies to prevent or treat complications. Incentive spirometry is designed to mimic natural sighing or yawning by encouraging the patient to take long, slow, deep breaths. This decreases pleural pressure, promoting increased lung expansion and better gas exchange. When the procedure is repeated on a regular basis, atelectasis may be prevented or reversed.

8. Yoga

Yoga is popularly understood to be a program of physical exercises (asana) and breathing exercises (pranayama). Yoga training aids in toning up of peripheral muscles, relaxing chest muscles and improving lung expansion, increasing respiratory stamina, raising energy levels and calming the body and mind. Efficient use of shoulder, thoracic and abdominal muscles can help in effective lung emptying during exhalation reducing dynamic hyper-inflation.

9. Staying hydrated

Getting enough water is as important for the lungs as it is for the rest of your body. Staying well hydrated by taking in fluids throughout the day helps keep the mucosal linings in the lungs thin. This thinner lining helps the lungs function better.

10. Diet

There is evidence that antioxidant rich foods (leafy green vegetables) are good for your lungs. Consumption of cruciferous vegetables (broccoli, cabbage, cauliflower, kale) reduces the risk of developing lung cancer.

Lung Transplantation

Lung transplantation has been used as a successful therapeutic intervention for a variety of end-stage pulmonary parenchymal and vascular diseases over the past 25 years. Advances in donor and recipient selection, surgical technique, and postoperative management have improved early survival. The criteria for use of either isolated lung transplantation or heart-lung transplantation continue to be defined, with the role of heart-lung transplantation lessening over the past decade.

General guidance for candidate selection for lung transplantation

Physicians evaluating patients for lung transplantation should ensure that the patient has received or is receiving maximum, optimal medical therapy for his disease but nevertheless has declining function. In general, candidates should have chronic disease for which no further medical or surgical therapy is available and survival is limited; lung transplantation is rarely an option for acutely, critically ill patients. Comorbid medical conditions should also be optimally treated in transplant candidates.

Older patients have a significantly worse survival rate than younger patients. The following guidelines are suggested.

Age limits
- Heart-lung transplants
  ~ 55 years
- Single lung transplants
  ~ 65 years
- Bilateral lung transplants
  ~ 60 years

General indications for lung transplantation

End stage pulmonary parenchymal and/or vascular disease:
- Projected life expectancy < 2 years
- NYHA class III or IV functional level
- Rehabilitation potential
- Disease-specific mortality exceeding transplant-specific mortality over 1–2 years

Disease-specific indications for lung transplantation

Obstructive lung disease—a BODE index of 7–10
- Chronic obstructive pulmonary disease
- α_1 Antitrypsin deficiency

Restrictive lung disease
- Idiopathic pulmonary fibrosis—FVC < 50% predicted, PaO_2< 50 mmHg, $PaCO_2$> 45 mmHg
  Pulmonary artery hypertension
  No response to steroid therapy
- Interstitial lung disease
  Sarcoidosis

Desquamative interstitial pneumonitis

Lymphangioleiomyomatosis
  Chemotherapy or radiation therapy related fibrosis
  Collagen vascular disorders with primarily pulmonary involvement
  Eosinophilic granuloma or histiocytosis X
  Alveolar microlithiasis

Septic lung disease
- Cystic fibrosis: FEV_1 <30% predicted, FVC ≤ 40% predicted, PaO_2 <60 mmHg, room air
  bilateral bronchiectasis

Hypogammaglobulinemia

Postinfectious (childhood measles, pertussis, postpneumonia, or tuberculosis)

  Immotile cilia syndrome—Kartagener's syndrome

  Allergic bronchopulmonary aspergillosis

* Pulmonary vascular disease

    Primary pulmonary hypertension—symptomatic disease

Eisenmenger's syndrome

Indications for specific lung transplant procedures

Single lung transplantation (SLT)

* Obstructive lung disease
* Restrictive lung disease
* Unilateral septic lung disease
* Primary pulmonary hypertension
* Eisenmenger's syndrome with a correctable shunt defect

Double lung transplantation (DLT)

* Obstructive lung disease (patient < 50 years old)
* Bilateral septic lung disease
* Primary pulmonary hypertension
* Eisenmenger's syndrome with a correctable shunt defect

Combined heart-lung transplantation (HLT)

* Refractory right ventricular end-diastolic dysfunction (RVEDP < 15 mmHg)
* Significant coronary artery disease, not amenable to non-surgical interventions
* Eisenmenger's syndrome with a irreparable shunt defect

Characteristics of a suitable lung donor

Age < 60 years

Cigarette smoking < 30 pack years

No significant prior thoracic surgery on the side of the donor lung

Normal chest radiograph of the donor lung

Adequate gas exchange of the donor lung

* PaO_2 > 300 mmHg on FIO_2 1.0, PEEP ≥ 5 cm
* PVO_2 > 450 mmHg on FIO_2 1.0, PEEP ≥ 5 cm

Bronchoscopic evaluation demonstrating absence of mucosal inflammation

No significant pulmonary trauma or anatomic abnormalities

Absolute contraindications for lung transplantation	Relative contraindications for lung transplantation
• Malignancy in the last 2 years, with the exception of cutaneous squamous and basal cell tumors. After lung malignancy, the recipient should wait for 5 years before receiving transplant.	• Age older than 65 years. If the donor is old, the outcome of lung transplant is inferior. Although there cannot be endorsement of an upper age limit as an absolute contraindication
• Untreatable advanced dysfunction of another major organ system (e.g. heart, liver, or kidney). Coronary heart disease which cannot be treated by routine standard medical procedures is	• Critical or unstable clinical conditions (e.g. shock, mechanical ventilation or extra-corporeal membrane oxygenation).

a contraindication to lung transplant but heart-lung transplantation could be considered in highly selected cases.

- Non-curable chronic extrapulmonary infection including chronic active viral hepatitis B, hepatitis C, and human immunodeficiency virus.

- Significant chest wall/spinal deformity

- Documented non-adherence or inability to follow through with medical therapy or office follow-up, or both.

- Untreatable psychiatric or psychologic condition associated with the inability to cooperate or comply with medical therapy.

- Absence of a consistent or reliable social support system.

- Substance addiction (e.g. alcohol, tobacco, or narcotics) that is either active or within the last 6 months.

- Severely limited functional status with poor rehabilitation potential.

- Colonization with highly resistant or highly virulent bacteria, fungi, or mycobacteria.

- Severe obesity defined as a body mass index (BMI) exceeding 30 kg/m^2.

- Severe or symptomatic osteoporosis.

- Mechanical ventilation. The selection process for lung transplant should be carefully done, candidates on mechanical ventilation without acute or chronic lung problems and willing to cooperate in the rehabilitation process.

- Other medical conditions that have not resulted in end-stage organ damage, such as diabetes mellitus, systemic hypertension, peptic ulcer disease, or gastroesophageal reflux should be optimally treated before transplantation. Patients with coronary artery disease may undergo percutaneous intervention before transplantation or coronary artery bypass grafting concurrent with the procedure.

Contraindications to lung transplantation

Absolute contraindications

- Bone marrow failure
- Hepatic cirrhosis
- Active malignancy precluding long-term survival
- Other life limiting conditions

Relative contraindications

- Physiological age

> 65 years for single-lung transplantation

> 60 years for double-lung transplantation

> 55 years for heart-lung transplantation

  - Psychosocial instability
  - Tobacco use within 6 months
  - Weight outside acceptable range (obesity or cachexia)
  - Prednisone use > 20 mg/day or 40 mg q.o.d.
  - Mechanical ventilation
  - Intrinsic renal disease
  - Significant peripheral vascular disease

- Symptomatic osteoporosis
- Severe chest wall deformity
- Sputum with panresistant bacteria or aspergillus
- Active hepatitis B or C infection

Recipient evaluation for lung transplantation

- Hematology

Complete blood count with differential, platelet count, PT, PTT, ESR

- Chemistry

Na, K, Cl, CO_2, BUN, Cr, glucose, osmolality, uric acid, Ca, P, Mg, total protein, albumin, globulin, amylase, bilirubin (direct, indirect), alkaline phosphatase, SGOT, SGPT, LDH, CPK, triglycerides, cholesterol, HDL/LDL

- Renal function

Urinalysis, 24 hr for calcium and creatinine

- Endocrine

TSH, LH, FSH, vitamin D, testosterone (males), estradiol (females)

- Infectious disease

Sputum (Gram's stain, C&S, fungal smear and culture, AFB smear and culture), CMV, hepatitis B (antigen/antibody), hepatitis C, herpes, varicella, EBV, HIV, rapid plasma regain, toxoplasma PPD, mumps, candida skin tests

- Immunology

ABO blood type and crossmatch, MHC typing, HLA sensitization (PRA screen)

- Radiology

Chest radiograph (AP, lateral), high resolution CT scan, quantitative V/Q scan, quantitative bone density, abdominal ultrasonography, sinus CT

- Cardiology

ECG, echocardiogram with pulse Doppler imaging, right heart catheterization, left heart catheterization

- Pulmonary

Pulmonary function tests (spirometry, lung volumes, DLCO), Baird level II exercise test

Summary

Significant progress has been made in the development of techniques of lung transplantation for all types of end-stage pulmonary diseases. Isolated lung transplantation has been applied with the increasing success to the entire group of patients, including those with pulmonary vascular disease. A shortage of donor organs, however, remains the most significant obstacle to the wider use of this method of treatment. Surgical mortality is 10 to 15 percent, slightly lower for SLT, and slightly higher for DLT and HLT. Functional results in the survivors of the operation are excellent. Infection remains a significant source of morbidity and mortality in both the early and late postoperative periods. However, the most significant impediment to long-term survival is the development of chronic rejection in the lung allograft, manifested as bronchiolitis obliterans syndrome, in half of the patients in 5 years after transplantation. Further measures to prevent or treat this malady are critical to improving long-term survival rates following lung transplantation.

Further Reading

1. American Journal of Respiratory and Critical Care Medicine, Volume 158, Pages 335–9.

2. Fishman's Pulmonary Diseases and Disorders, 4th edition, Volume 2.

3. http://lungfoundation.com.au/lung-health

4. http://www.empowher.com/lung-conditions/content/8-tips-help-prevent-lung-disease

5. http://www.health.com/health/gallery

6. http://www.lung.org/lung-health-and-diseases/protecting-your-lungs

7. https://www.lung.ca/lung-health/prevent-lung-disease

8. https://www.rush.edu/health-wellness/discover-health/keeping-your-lungs-healthy

9. Murray and Nadel's Textbook of Respiratory Medicine, 5th edition, Volume 2.

Treatment of Heart and Lung Failure

Nandkishore Kapadia

INTRODUCTION

Heart failure affects 23 million people worldwide with more than 10 million in India. Medical therapy such as diuretics, ACE inhibitors and maximum tolerable doses of beta blockers is very effective. However, in non-responders with terminal heart failure intra-aortic balloon pump, permanent left and right heart support devices and heart transplant may be the only curative therapy. Number of donors is insufficient to meet demand. International Society for Heart and Lung Transplantation (ISHLT) registry has reported 89,000 heart transplants worldwide.

History

First heart transplant was done by Christian Bernard in South Africa *on 3rd December 1967, patient lived 18 days.*

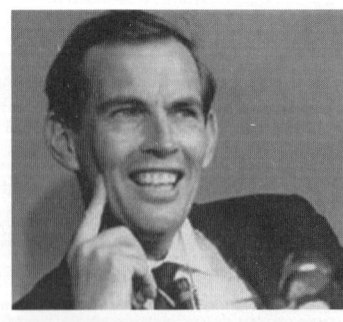

Dr *Norman Shumway* did first successful heart transplant in USA. Dr P K Sen did first heart transplant in India at KEM Mumbai in 1968. Cyclosporine discovery (1983), improved results of heart transplant. *Dr Venogopal* (AIIMS

Delhi) did first successful heart transplantation in India (1994). First heart transplant in child was done by KM Cherian (Chennai: June 2009). Mumbai witnessed first successful heart transplant in August 2015. Tamil Nadu is leader in organising organ sharing network. 290 heart transplant were done in Tamil Nadu between October 2008 and December 2016 and 94 elsewhere in India totalling 384.

Terminal Heart Failure

These patients are in New York Heart Association (NYHA) Class III and IV.

Dilated cardiomyopathy

Ischemic cardiomyopathy

Restrictive cardiomyopathy

Hypertrophic cardiomyopathy

Complex congenital heart disease

Indications for heart transplantation Causes for terminal heart failure are indications for heart transplant: Stage D heart failure due to any cause with preserved end-organs (lungs, kidney and liver).

Pre-transplantation evaluation is done by: Exercise capacity as assessed by peak VO_2 (VO_{2max}): Considered gold standard, if <14 mL/min/kg, heart transplant indicated.

Heart Transplant Contraindications

I. Irreversible renal failure with Cr >2

II. Irreversible liver disease

III. Advanced lung disease

IV. Pulmonary hypertension (PVR > 5)

V. Solid organ or hematologic malignancy

Indian network of organ sharing (NOTTO SOTTO ROTTO ZTCC), Regional net working organization gives highest status to seriously ill hospital patients on inotropic drugs or mechanical circulatory support (LVAD, ECMO). Others are on routine wait list.

Management of Patients on the Waiting List

Pharmacotherapy

- Diuretics, ACE inhibitors, beta blockers
- **Inotropic therapy:** Dobutamine and milrinone, are used to help maintain end-organ function.

Mechanical Circulatory Support as Bridge to Heart Transplant

Mechanical circulatory support is by ECMO, VAD, tandem heart. Approximately, 8% of these patients die awaiting suitable allograft.

Rejection: It is T-lymphocyte event, although humoral with preformed antibodies to human leukocyte antigens (HLA) result immediate rejection.

Immunosuppression regimens

Induction therapy reduces acute rejection: ATGAM, thymoglobulin, basiliximab.

Maintenance therapy consists of combination, of cyclosporine or tacrolimus, mycopheolate, steroids, first two agents cause kidney damage.

Immunosuppression drug level monitoring

Immunosuppressive agent	Therapeutic level
Cyclosporine (ng/ml)	180–200
Tacrolimus (ng/ml)	10–20

Surveillance of Rejection

Done by Endo-myocardial biopsy, echocardiography and donor derived antibody.

Late Complications

Major causes of late morbidity and mortality are infections, chronic kidney disease, cardiac allograft vasculopathy (CAV) and malignancy.

Coronary artery vasculopathy (CAV)

Coronary vasculopathy develops in 30% to 40% of heart transplant recipients within 5 years, may need bypass surgery or stenting.

Infectious complications

Bacteria and viruses account for 80% of severe infections after heart transplant. The cytomegalovirus infection (CMV), toxoplasmosis, tuberculosis occur late.

- **Renal dysfunction:** Tacrolimus and cyclosporine blood levels is critically important to limit progressive decline in kidney function.
- **Malignancy:** Malignancy risk is estimated at 1% to 2% per years.

Conclusions

Survival and quality of life after heart transplantation is excellent. One year survival rate is 90%, 5-year is 70% and 20% survive for 20 years.

Respiratory Failure

Introduction: Respiratory failure results from inadequate gas exchange by lungs due to dysfunction of one or more essential components of respiratory system mostly failure of alveolar–capillary units. Drop in the oxygen and a rise in arterial carbon dioxide are highly characteristics.

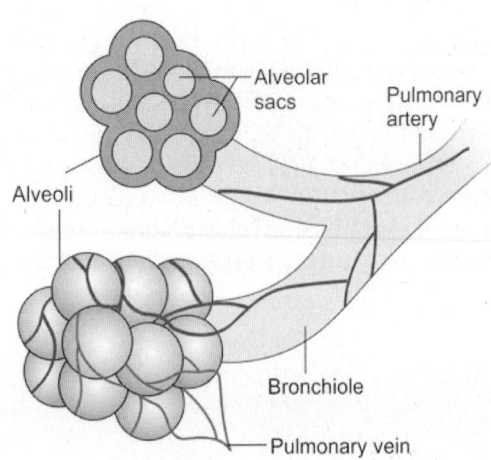

Fig. 4.1: Respiratory system

Classification of Respiratory Failure

Type I or Hypoxemic (PaO$_2$ <60): *Failure of oxygen exchange* refractory to supplemental oxygen

Type II Hypercapnic (PaCO$_2$ >45): *Failure to remove carbon dioxide.*

Type III: *Perioperative respiratory failure.* Increased atelectasis.

Type IV: Following resuscitation for shock.

Acute Respiratory Failure: Management

It is treated by ventilatory support with or without tracheostomy. Acute respiratory syndrome not a part of multiorgan dysfunction carries a reasonable prognosis. If this fails, they may require temporary support by artificial lungs, namely extra corporeal membrane oxygenation (ECMO) or nova lung.

Patients not amenable to medical or ventilatory therapy are candidates for lung transplant.

Indications of Lung Transplant

1. Chronic obstructive lung disease.
2. Cystic fibrosis/bronchiectatic diseases.
3. Idiopathic pulmonary fibrosis.
4. Primary pulmonary hypertension.
5. Pulmonary hypertension due to congenital heart disease (Eisenmenger's syndrome).

Listing of Patients for Lung Transplant and Pre-Transplant Work up

Donor Selection

Ideal lung donor should be non-smoker < 55 years, without lung contusion, pulmonary oedema, pulmonary tuberculosis, cancer, septicaemia, hepatitis A, B , C , HIV negative, with arterial PO$_2$ > 400 and pCO$_2$ < 40 on 100% oxygen on ventilator. All donors should have CT scan of chest besides chest X-ray. Physical examination of lungs by an experienced trans-plant surgeon is the best method to assess for lung injury and transplant suitability.

Harvesting of Lungs

Cardioplegia and pneumoplegia are given (Perfadex, THAM, prostacycline), inflated lungs are transported in ice box. Lung transplant must be over within 4 hours.

Single or Double Lung Transplant

Depends on pathology and indication. Double lungs transplant gives superior results but immediate morbidity is high.

Surgical Techniques

Main bronchus is anastomosed followed by pulmonary artery and vein. Mostly no heart lung machine required. Immediately after lung transplant, bronchoscopy is done to clear secretions.

Immunosuppression and Prophylaxis

- Induction with basiliximab and methyl-prednisolone.
- Maintenance with cyclosporine, tacrolimus, mycophenolate, prednisolone.
- *Pneumocystis carinii* pneumonia (PCP) and CMV prophylaxis for 6 months and 3 months respectively.

Complications

- **Fatal complications:** Failure of lung graft requiring ECMO, prolonged ventilation, lung infection bacterial, viral, fungal, mycobacterial carry high mortality.
- **Rejection is common:** Rejection surveillance is done with chest X-ray, bronchoscopy and BAL/biopsy.

Survival

- 1-year survival < 80%.
- 5-year survival < 50%.

Heart and Lung Transplant

Anvay Mulay, Sandeep Sinha, Santosh Sorate

The aim of coordinator is to promote awareness in the community about organ donation. The coordinators should reach out to actively encourage and increase awareness of coexisting issues surrounding organ and tissue donation among health professionals of all disciplines.

Irrespective of their organization to which the coordinators are attached, they have unwritten power to approach donor family, recipient family, professionals, administrative and state authorities.

They are "NARAD MUNI" of Organ Donation and Transplant program! Master of communication. Therefore, have vital duties and moral responsibilities.

Clinical coordinator should have good knowledge of medicine and the discipline, which coordinator is working for. They should also have understanding of law and administration, communication skills. Along with social coordinators they play a key role in screening, arranging, both recipient as well as donor. Planning the logistic of retrieving the organs and time bound scheduling of harvesting, transporting safely, coordinators are backbone of the program.

Social coordinators are broadly three types, according to their organizational attachment. Accordingly, the scope of their work expands beyond their primary aim of propagating organ donation.

Those social workers who work with transplant teams are called transplant social coordinators.

What are expectations from coordinators? What basics coordinator must know as they start working in transplant team?

There are some basic things which all coordinators must know across the sector and discipline. There are some specialized things in addition that transplant coordinators should know and are expected to do. Interestingly as one moves from social coordinator to transplant social coordinator, the scope of duties, expectations and in-depth knowledge of the program increases.

Authorities and coordinators are advised that changes in guidelines and protocols at institutions and state level take place all the time and over and over, therefore should update themselves regularly.

The coordinators for transplant should promote cadaveric organ donation program for solid and hollow organs than live donor program. This is the need of the time.

Transplant social coordinators should have knowledge about medicine and Govt. rules, regulations and laws of the state regarding organ donation, their distribution of solid organ for transplant.

The social coordinator should concentrate on counselling of donor family for organ donation. Promoting declaration of death as brain dead among professionals and hospital administrators.

This is extremely vital in cadaveric organ donation program.

Who can donate which organ is a domain of the expert in that discipline or faculty. The types of organs and tissues that can be donated will depend on the donor criteria and also to some extent recipient critical status.

At the time of potential organ donor referral, social coordinator should have information of donor:

1. Cause of death,
2. Age of the donor,
3. Past medical history like diabetes, hypertension, CKD, genetic or familial condition, smoker, major operation, etc.
4. Current status of the organs and tissues to be retrieved.

Organ Donation After Brain Death

Brain dead patient can donate almost all essential and vital organs heart, lung, liver, kidney, pancreas, stomach, intestine, bone, eyes, skin.

Patients who have suffered permanent loss of brain function (brain death) but still have functioning cardiovascular system, are potential donors of these organs.

Organ donation is possible only in the event of ICU or emergency department death. They are still maintained by mechanical ventilation and their circulatory system well supported.

Organ donation cannot take place until death has been confirmed and authorization has been obtained. Also after cessation of circulation in a brain-dead patient, the diseased is not eligible to donate organs like heart, lung, liver and kidney.

Depending upon the donor criteria as mentioned above each diseased is considered individually but broadly and most importantly:

1. The patient must have suffered irreversible loss of brain function (brain death)
2. Maintained on a ventilator with well-supported intact circulation

Exclusion criteria for organ donation social coordinators must know.

There are relative exclusion criteria for each organ separately but in general:

1. Human immunodeficiency virus (HIV)
2. Current neoplastic disease other than primary brain tumors and non-malignant skin cancers.

Such a donor who is willing to donate organ should be screened by/examined by specialized doctors who are authorized.

Such experts then conduct apnea test. This is done after confirmed consent for organ donation. This is repeated after the interval of minimum 6 hours.

During the apnea tests or immediately after, the donors may become unstable and deteriorate fast, therefore for organs like heart, lung, liver, kidney, the coordinators should inform the authorities about the potential donor at earliest to local authorities like ZTCC/SOTTO/ROTTO.

This allows adequate time, to find the appropriate recipient according to the rules of priority set by them.

This also gives time for logistic working, arranging, travelling arrangements, conducting necessary tests to see the current status of the organ. In short, the recipient team can prepare for the retrieval and confirm to the state authorities accordingly without wasting time. This also allows the heart and lung team in coordination with donor medical team to stabilize the donor and perform some key tests like 2D echo, bronchoscopy, CT scan if and whenever necessary.

In this communication between donor family—hospital and medical staff—state authorities who distribute the organs—recipient medical staff and clinical coordinator—recipient family—recipient hospital/transplant center, arrangements for transporting the organ-police authorities and green corridor ... the transplant social coordinator is an anchor.

Social and clinical coordinators have to be multifaceted, multipurpose, skillful communicators. They are responsible for smooth, flawless and ethical, co-ordination between various teams, authorities, helping recipient and donor family.

They are one-point contact between coordinators, common man, professionals and bureaucrats.

The coordinators are vital to transplant program. They play key role in preoperative, intraoperative and postoperative heart transplant patient.

Getting the registration of recipients. Helping and arranging the finance from charity and individuals. Ensuring the organ for them by propagating the need for donating organs among the community.

Sentence can start transplant social coordinators are the first one to get the information of likelihood of potential or probable organ donation. They get this information from the state authorities who distribute the organs.

It is the responsibility of the social coordinators of donor and state organ distribution authority to confirm the brain death certification from authorized experts. Without this confirmation, state authority should not allocate the organ to transplant teams.

Transplant coordinator and transplant team should confirm this once again before proceeding for retrieval of organs.

Social transplant coordinator alerts clinical transplant coordinator and collect the information of donor, donor hospital, and medical team treating the donor. Social coordinator try to find logistic of approaching and retrieving the organ along with the other transplant teams. All the time keeping in touch with donor coordinator, state authorities and hospital administration.

Clinical coordinator finds out the details of the donor. At the time of potential donor referral, it is helpful to have patient charts available, as additional information may be required by the transplant team.

- Patient's name and gender
- Age and date of birth
- Body weight
- Blood group
- Cause of death
- Status of brain death testing (time of death, if available)
- Potential exclusion criteria (if known)
- Past medical history
- Blood results (if available)
- Course of treatment throughout admission
- Family details and needs (e.g. the request for the handover of the body before specific time)

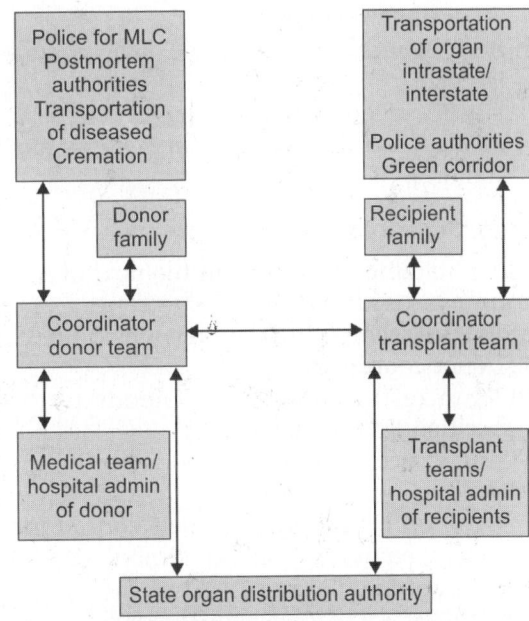

Fig. 5.1: MSW during cadaver transplant

Specific Organ Criteria

Variations in age limits apply to all solid organs for donation. These are current general age limits for heart and lung. However, these limits are guidelines only.

- Heart donor—age up to 60 years
- Heart/lung and single lung donor—age up to 65 years.

To understand the current status and the condition of the organ for its usability, more information is needed.

For Heart Donors

1. ABG and serum electrolytes.
2. ECG
3. X-ray chest
4. CBC, if WBC high/fever—procalcitonin
5. 2D echo./TEE
6. Serum creatinine
7. Trop T, Trop I, CKMB in case of chest trauma
8. CAG in selected patients

For Lung Donors

1. FIO_2 and PO_2
2. ABG, serum electrolytes
3. X-ray chest

4. CT scan if possible
5. Body weight and height. Chest circumference
6. History of smoking/TB
7. Bronchoscopy if sputum of BAL—gram staining.

Donor Screening

After obtaining consent from the next of kin, blood can be drawn for tissue typing and serology screening. It is the responsibility of the donor coordinator to:

• Organize transport of the bloods to the specified testing facility
• Give advice on how the bloods need to be labelled and transported.

All blood tubes require labels containing the donors name, unit record number, date of birth, time and date the blood was drawn.

Please see below for general donor screening requirements.

Serology tests: Serology tests have to be done on the blood which is collected on admission of the donor. The sample required is pre-dilutional/transfusion sample. If unobtainable, then serology can be collected in standard 2 × 8 ml-serum clot activator tubes.

• HIV I and II
• HIV I antibody
• Hepatitis B sAg
• Hepatitis B sAb
• Hepatitis B Core Ab
• Hepatitis C sAb
• CMV (IgG)
• EBV

Tissue typing: Tissue typing is required for crossmatching of thoracic and abdominal organs and allocation of kidneys. The tubes required 8–18 × 10 ml ACD tubes (depending upon blood group).

Blood group: Blood group for ABO, Rhesus factor and antibody screen will also be required prior to sending tissue-typing samples.

Blood group A or AB may require blood group subtyping to determine the A1 or A2 status. The donor coordinator will facilitate this process if required.

These tests should be done as soon as possible to expedite the process and avoid lengthy wait for the donor family.

In case of **multi-organ donation utmost respect should be given to each organ and every team involved** for the cause. The team who arrives first should help in stabilizing the donor and wait for all the teams to be present, discuss plan and time line the harvesting schedule.

Evading these ethical duties and moral responsibilities is disrespect of lowest order, to the Nobel wish of donating organ by diseased family. This is the moral responsibility of social transplant coordinators.

Post-heart Transplant Medication and Precaution

Prashant Nair

INTRODUCTION

Cardiac transplantation, also called heart transplantation, has evolved into the treatment of choice for many people with severe heart failure who have severe symptoms despite maximum medical therapy. Improvement in the methods to suppress the immune system finally lead to improvement in survival. However, the number of heart transplant done in the world is stagnated at 5000 plus per year in contrast to 50000 recipients in waiting. This critical organ shortage means that health care providers must strictly evaluate who should receive a heart transplant.

A key to a successful heart transplant is working closely with a team. Here is a list of the team members and who should be a part of the transplant programme:

- Transplant cardiologist
- Transplant surgeon
- Transplant nurse coordinator
- Dietitian
- Social worker
- Financial admissions coordinator
- The patient

OUTCOME AFTER FIRST HEART TRANSPLANT

Survival: The survival rate is 85–90% at one year and 4% annual death rate. The three-year survival approaches 75 percent.

There is no difference in the survival among patients with congenital heart disease and other causes. One-year survival rate in people with congenital heart disease is 79 percent; at five years, the survival rate is 60 percent.

The various factors, which affect the outcome of the transplant, are enumerated here.

Recipient factors: Factors associated with an increased risk of death up to one year after transplantation include:

- Preoperative need for artificial breathing support (ventilator)
- If the heart transplantation is the second one for the recipient
- Heart conditions other than coronary artery disease or cardiomyopathy
- Preoperative need for heart function assistance with a ventricular assist device
- Being female
- Being underweight or obese

Donor factors: A variety of donor factors affect the early outcomes:

- A female donor is associated with increased one-year mortality.
- The age of the donor heart does not affect long-term survival, although transplant coronary artery disease is increased in hearts from donors over 40 years of age due to the presence of narrowing in the coronary arteries.
- Significant thickening of the left ventricle (left ventricular hypertrophy) in the donor heart is associated with poorer outcomes compared with a heart without thickening.

- Elevated blood levels of troponin I and T in the donor, which are markers of heart muscle damage, increase the risk of early heart failure.

Causes of death: There are four major causes of death after cardiac transplantation, which occur at different times:
- Sudden (acute) rejection
- Infections other than cytomegalovirus
- Artery disease in the transplanted heart vessels (allograft vasculopathy)
- Lymphoma and other malignancies.

Early mortality: Cardiac transplant recipients have an average of one to three episodes of rejection in the first year after transplantation. The incidence of acute rejection is common in the first 50–80% which is high. Thereafter the incidence decreases. The cause of death in the first year is acute rejection (18%) and infection (22%).

Late mortality: Rejection is less common after the first year, and by four to five years after transplantation, less than 10 percent of deaths are the result of rejection.

However, development of rapidly progressing coronary artery disease in the arteries of the transplanted heart (called allograft vasculopathy), becomes one of the most common causes of death by five years. The number of fatal cancers increases over time as well.

Infections

Infections remain a significant cause of death after the first year. These infections are the result of a weakened immune system, and can develop from common bacteria and viruses in the community or from uncommon infections.

Post-transplant lymphoproliferative disease (PTLD)—is a type of cancer that occurs in patients who use immunosuppressive medications. PTLD includes non-Hodgkin lymphoma. Most cases of PTLD occur in the first year after transplant. Among patients who develop lymphoma, the overall survival rates are between 25 and 35 percent at five years.

How is the Transplant Heart Different from Original Heart?

The transplanted heart is said to be denervated. When the heart is removed from the donor, the nerves to the heart are cut and the nervous system is "disconnected." During transplant surgery, the transplanted heart is not connected to the external nervous system. Although the transplanted heart will beat adequately, there is no connection to external nerves that will affect the heart rate. The heart transplant recipient is said to have a denervated heart. Although most heart transplant recipients have near normal function of the transplanted heart, there are some differences when the heart is denervated.

- Heart transplant recipients usually do not have chest pain (angina) if the blood flow through the coronary arteries is decreased. Patients with heart transplant do not have chest pain but will have fatigue, difficulty in breathing and inability to exercise.
- Heart transplant recipients have a faster resting heart rate, approximately 100 beats per minute.
- The heart rate of a denervated heart will not increase as quickly with exercise. Some patients may become mildly lightheaded or dizzy if they move around or change positions quickly. Because the transplanted heart is denervated, the patient will need to take some time to warm up before exercising. This will help to gradually increase your heart rate. Likewise, it will need to take several minutes to cool down after exercising. This will help the heart rate slowly return to normal. It may also be helpful for the patient to pump their legs and rotate the ankles several times before getting out of bed or out of a chair.

Immunosuppression

Heart transplant recipients require antirejection medications to suppress their immune system so that the transplanted heart is not rejected. Because the immune system is suppressed by these medications, transplant recipients are always at risk for infection. This risk is highest in the first three to six months after transplant.

Infections occur when higher immuno-suppression is given. If patient is doing well and has a good function of the transplanted heart, and have not had any episodes of rejection, the level of immunosuppression after a few months may slowly be lowered. Using less immunosuppression, when possible, will help minimize your risk of infection.

Stay Healthy

There are many ways to stay healthy after heart transplant and avoid infections. The following guidelines are commonly recommended for transplant recipients. The patient should discuss how to prevent the risk of infection with the transplant team. Know your center's specific guidelines.

Handwashing

- The hand should be washed properly with soap and water. Be sure to scrub between your fingers and under the nails. Waterless liquid soaps and gels can also be used when there is no visible dirt on the hands. These products are convenient to carry with in a purse or pocket. One must wash their hands well before eating and preparing food, after going to the bathroom, after changing diapers, and after playing with pets.
- Encourage any family and friends who are in contact to practice good handwashing techniques.
- Wash hands well before caring for any wounds or doing any dressing changes. Report any changes in the wound (increased redness, swelling, or drainage) to your transplant coordinator.
- Avoid putting fingers or hands in or near the mouth, particularly if they are not washed recently.

Contacts

- The patients should not interact with other people with cold and flu.
- Avoid crowds, particularly when in a closed area like an indoor shopping mall, during cold and flu season or when you are highly immunosuppressed.

- Do not share eating utensils, cups, glasses or toothbrushes with others since many viral illnesses are spread through saliva and mucous.
- Do not share razors, nail clippers or other manicure equipment.

Immunosuppression Levels

The level of anti-rejection medicine in the blood is monitored very closely after transplant. It is important that the level that is high enough to prevent rejection, but not so high that one develops infections easily. The level of the anti-rejection medicine is highest during the first three to six months after transplant. If one does not have rejection and if the heart is working well, the dose of medications level will be decreased slowly over time. If there is rejection, the immuno-suppression level will be increased. The doses of anti-rejection medications may change frequently depending on if one is experiencing rejection or infection.

Nutrition

A healthy diet is one that is made up of fruits, vegetables, whole grains, and low fat or fat free milk and milk products. It also includes lean meats, poultry, fish, eggs, nuts, and beans. A healthy diet should be low in saturated fats, trans fat, salt, added sugar, and cholesterol. Good nutrition is an important part of a complete recovery following heart transplant. As one recovers, the body has increased nutritional needs for wound healing, to regain any weight lost due to heart disease and the stress of surgery, and to help the body fight infection. After heart transplant, patients need a diet high in calories and protein to rebuild muscle tissue and restore protein levels. Dietary requirements are different for everyone, so the dietician will need to be met with to discuss specific nutritional and caloric needs and any dietary restrictions one may need. For a while after surgery, most patients will need to increase calories as well as calcium and protein intake. During the first few weeks after transplant, some patients have trouble eating due to loss of appetite, feeling full or nauseated, or because they have changes in taste. This is quite common and will resolve over time as patients recover and activity increases. If one has a poor appetite, try to eat several small meals a day, snack between meals on high calorie and high protein foods, and/or drink higher calorie liquids such as milk or juice rather than water.

Activity

Exercise improves one's overall health. It makes the patient feel better and can help control stress. Regular exercise can help maintain a weight that is right for the patient. It can also help prevent bone disease (osteoporosis). Any form of exercise is beneficial. It is common to feel tired or weak as one recovers from heart transplant. If one has been hospitalized for a long time before or after the transplant, one may have lost some muscle mass from prolonged bed rest. One may also find that the sleep pattern is disturbed. Regular exercise and good nutrition will help one get back to a more active routine. Transplant recipients should discuss how to start an exercise program with their doctor and transplant team so that a safe exercise plan can be developed.

Cardiac rehabilitation can be very helpful following heart transplant. These programs help heart transplant patients gradually and safely increase their activity level. Cardiac rehabilitation programs teach patients how to exercise safely after heart transplant and can also help increase a patient's confidence in their ability to exercise.

For the first six months after transplant, one may be advised to avoid any strenuous activity, heavy lifting, or more intensive exercise programs. Walking is the best form of exercise after transplant. Remember that the patient will also need several minutes to warm up and cool down because the transplanted heart is denervated. Most centers recommend that to avoid any activities or sports with a high risk of injury like football, wrestling, skiing, water skiing, or motorcycling. To be healthy and fit is an important goal, but using common sense to reach this goal is just as important. The patient should stop exercising immediately if they experience the following while exercising:

- Pain or pressure in your chest, neck or jaw
- Intense fatigue that is not related to a lack of sleep
- Unusual shortness of breath
- Dizziness or light-headedness during or after exercise
- A continuing rapid or irregular heart rate during or after exercise

Returning to School or Work Post-heart Transplant

Recipients return to work or school at various times after recovery from transplant surgery. The return depends on the extent of the illness before transplant, recovery time, complications, and the type of work that is done. Most patients are ready to return to work or school within three months after transplant. When possible, it can be helpful to return to work or school on a part-time basis. One can gradually increase the hours as the energy and strength improves.

Driving

Most transplant recipients can resume driving within four to six weeks after transplant, depending on their recovery period, complications, and medications. The patient's reflexes and judgment may be affected from being ill, from having a lengthy hospitalization, or by some medications. It is best to discuss this issue with the doctor and coordinator before getting behind the wheel. It is a good idea to practice driving in an open lot or away from other traffic for the first time as one gets used to driving again. It may be helpful to have another licensed driver in the car for the first few times. When driving or in a car, always wear a seat belt. If the chest is still sore, padding their chest with a towel or small pillow will help cushion the incision from the seat belt. The seat belt will provide a safe restraint in case of an accident.

Travelling

As one recovers and returns to a more normal routine, one may consider travelling or going on a vacation. Some centers recommend waiting for 6 to 12 months before taking an extended vacation, particularly one that may be farther away from major hospitals or transplant centers. If one is planning a vacation, one may be advised to have the routine blood tests taken a few weeks before the travel. If one is traveling to a different time zone the patient needs to how to adjust the medication times. Before one leaves, the patient should be sure to know where the closest hospital and/or transplant center is located in case of an emergency. The patient should take enough medication to last the entire trip plus some extra in case the trip is extended. If one is travelling to a foreign country one may need a letter from the transplant team that lists all the medications. Some transplant programs give patients an antibiotic to take with them in case they develop an infection and do not have access to a pharmacy. Taking extra medications and packing them in a different bag may also be helpful if the airline misplace the luggage. Travel to third world countries to be avoided in patients with immunosuppression. The risk of getting infections in these areas is high and appropriate healthcare may not be available. Additionally, some foreign travel may require immunizations that are not safe for patients who are immunosuppressed, such as measles and smallpox.

Sexual Activity

Before transplant, many patients experience a decreased desire (libido) to have sex or are unable to have sex (impotence) because of health problems and activity limitations. After transplant, both men and women often find that their desire and ability to have sex returns. It is better to wait for 8 weeks after transplant to resume sexual activity. How quickly one is ready to have sex after transplant depends on how the patient feels. There are many reasons why patients can have problems with sexual activity. Difficulties could be from complications related to their original cardiac disease, medications, or problems in their relationship with their partners. When one is ready to resume sexual activity, it may be helpful to discuss any concerns the patient has with their partners.

Cornea, Skin, Hand and Body Donation

Eye Donation

Kamaxi Bhate

INTRODUCTION

India has the largest number of blind people in the world. More than 12 million Indians are without eyesight—that is, one in a hundred Indians are blind. Out of these, three million have corneal blindness. Sixty percent of those with corneal blindness are children below the age of 12 years.

The problem of blindness in India is enormous. Sadly, our society is, by and large, blind to this problem. The societal blindness manifests itself in the form of indifference, insensitivity and ignorance.

Corneal blindness can be treated by replacing the damaged cornea with a donated healthy human cornea. The only source of human cornea is Eye Donation. Since a living person cannot donate his or her eye, human cornea can be sourced from the cadavers only.

What is Cornea?

Cornea is the transparent, dome-shaped window covering the front of the eye. It is a powerful refracting surface, providing two-thirds of the eye's focusing power. Like the crystal on a watch, this clear covering of the eye gives us a window to look through. Because there are no blood vessels in the cornea, it is normally clear and has a shiny surface. The cornea is extremely sensitive—there are more nerve endings in the cornea than anywhere else in the body.

Why is there Corneal Blindness?

Corneal blindness is seen mostly in poor countries, and among the poor in developing countries. The main causes of corneal failure worldwide are trachoma, vitamin A deficiency, herpes simplex and other types of infectious keratitis, injuries to the eye, and complications following surgery. These diseases and complications destroy the optical function of the cornea by scarring and opacification, and by stromal melting and thinning that cause surface topographic irregularity causing opacity and blindness.

History of Corneal Transplantation

The first successful transplant was by Vladimir Filatov, a Russian ophthalmologist who is considered to be the father of keratoplasty, performed the surgery in 1935 by utilising a human donor cornea from the eyeball stored in moist chamber at 4°C.

In response to the growing demand for human corneal tissue, the first eye bank for sight restoration was started in New York in 1944. Since then eye banking movement has spread worldwide. In India, the first eye bank was established in Madras in 1945.

What is an Eye Bank?

Eye Bank is an organisation which deals with the collection, storage and distribution of the donor cornea for the purpose of corneal grafting, research and supply of eye tissue to other eye banks for ophthalmic purposes. Comprehensive and detailed standards of eye banking have been formulated to assure consistency, quality, proficiency, and ethics in dealing with eye tissue for harvesting, transportation and research. *The functioning of eye banks is governed by the Human Organ Transplant Act (HOTA).*

Facts about eye donation—that the common people should know.

1. *All of us can be donors*: Almost anyone of any age and sex can pledge to donate eyes after death. This can be done even if the donor wears glasses, has cataract or has undergone eye surgery successfully. All that is needed is a clear, healthy cornea.

2. *Relatives are decision makers*: The eyes of the deceased can be donated whether he/she has pledged the eye during life or not. At the same time, eyes cannot be removed without the consent of the next of kin, even if the deceased has already pledge his eyes.

3. *Time is important*: The eyes have to be removed within **six hours** of death. The eye bank, which is nearest to the hospital, has to be informed immediately.

4. *Keep it moist*: Eye lids of the dead should be closed immediately after death. Head end should be elevated, fans should be switched off and a wet piece of cloth should be placed over the covered eyes. Antibiotic drops, if available, may be applied to keep the eye moist, so that the cornea does not dry up.

5. *Death at home*: In case of death being reported from a place other than a hospital, an eye bank team with a doctor/technician will reach the donor site including his or her home. No fee is charged to the family for eye donation.

6. *No scar*: Excising an eye takes only 15–20 minutes and leaves no scar or disfigurement of the face.

7. *You light up two lives!*: Two blind people can receive sight after eye donation from a single person.

8. *Speedy transplant*: On reaching the eye bank, the donated eyes are examined, processed and used for corneal transplant operation as early as possible.

9. *Anonymity*: The recipient of cornea will always remain anonymous but the donor's family should be satisfied knowing that the eyes have been used to restore the vision of a blind person[s].

10. *Eye donation is free and voluntary*: The donated eyes are never bought or sold. Eye donation offered is never refused.

11. *Eye donation is easy*: It is only one phone call away. Call the nearest eye bank on 1919 or 1053 or 104.

We can do it

India is a large country with a population of 125 million. There are more than 60,000 deaths per day. If 100% Indians decide to donate their eyes after death, all the corneal blind persons can get the eyesight in just 11 days! Even if 5 percent of the people donate eyes after death, we can achieve the same result in 220 days!

As Helen Keller, a legendary American who overcame her deafness and blindness to become one of the world's leading humanitarians, says, *There is no better way to thank God for your sight than by giving a helping hand to someone in the dark.* Here all of us have a chance to thank God enough by pledging our eyes to be donated after our death!

"Please turn off the lights, when you leave!" is a good energy-saving message we read in our offices and public buildings. For removing blindness in our society through eye donation, we should modify that message to read— *Please turn on the lights, whenever you leave!*

Skin Donation and Skin Banking

S Keswani

Background

Burns is considered as a neglected health crisis globally. More so in India—as the majority who get burnt are women and children, most of whom cannot afford the 'high-on-cost' burns treatment. In most of these cases there is high mortality and morbidity due to infection and dehydration at the burns site. With this as the background, there was a great need of establishing a skin bank in India to collect process and preserve human cadaver skin donated after death. The processed donor skin helps immensely in the treatment of extensive burns as a temporary dressing.

The RCBN Skin Bank (Rotary Club of Bombay North Skin Bank) started in November 2009 at National Burns Centre (NBC) with the help of Rotary Club of Bombay North and Rotary Club of Leiden, Amsterdam and technical collaboration with Euro Skin Bank, Amsterdam.

Concept of Skin Donation

Most of the mortality and morbidity can be prevented if these patients get a human skin covering on their burnt area. This covering stays for three-four weeks and by that time patient's own skin regenerates. It also reduces the pain due to burns. Thus, human skin acts as a life saver in these severely ill patients.

The Skin bank not only caters to National Burns Centre (NBC) requirement but it also caters to the whole nation as there is no other skin bank of such high quality in the country today.

Benefits of Donated Skin

1. Prevents infection
2. Reduces the pain
3. Improves immunity
4. Faster healing (so, reduced hospital stay and reduced cost of treatment)
5. Prevents heat loss
6. Prevents loss of body fluids

Facts and Figures

1. Skin can be donated within 6 hours of death.
2. Any one above the age of 18 years can donate skin, there is no upper age limit.
3. *Skin Donation Helpline*: 022 2779 3333
4. *Skin collection centre of RCBN skin bank*: BSES Hospital, Andheri
5. Only a thin layer is taken from legs, thighs and back.
6. *During harvesting*: No bleeding. No disfigurement.
7. No fees have to be paid for this service.
8. For grafting, no donor-recipient matching required. No blood matching or color matching required.

Contraindications

Skin cannot be donated if the donor has died of any of the following:

1. HIV/HBsAg/HCV/VDRL positive or any other viral infection
2. Jaundice

3. TB/pneumonia or related respiratory disorders.
4. Sepsis/bacteraemia or any kind of skin diseases/bed sores.
5. Skin cancer or any malignancy
6. Sexually transmitted diseases.
7. Varicose veins

Procedure

The skin harvesting procedure is simple.

1. Within 6 hours of death, relatives of the person/NGO/transplant coordinator can call the Skin Donation Helpline: 022 2779 3333
2. The Skin Bank team confirms the details of death (Death Certificate), contraindications, address, cremation/funeral timings, etc. over phone/WhatsApp.
3. Once confirmed, the skin bank team (doctor/biotechnologist and two nurses) will reach the house or hospital (wherever the deceased has been kept) within 2 hours of the call depending on the distance.
4. Once they reach the place, they explain the procedure and purpose of skin donation to the relatives, take a copy of the death certificate and get the consent form signed.
5. Thereafter the body is examined, cleaned and a thin layer of skin is harvested from both the legs, thighs, and the back with a special instrument called DERMATOME. Along with skin, blood sample is also collected from the deceased donor for checking for viral diseases.

6. After skin is harvested, the donor area is bandaged and no disfigurement or bleeding is noticed. This entire procedure takes only 45 minutes. Then, the donor's body is handed over to the next of kin. Finally, a certificate of Skin Donation and Thank you letter is given to the donor's relatives for this noble gesture.
7. The skin is preserved in a glycerol solution and is transported to the RCBN Skin Bank at National Burns Center, Airoli. The harvested skin is thereafter processed, checked for viral, bacterial and fungal infection and can be preserved for up to 5 years at the Skin Bank at 4–8 degree Celcius as per Euro Skin Bank protocols.
8. It is distributed to needy burns patients across the country at ambient temperatures upon official request by the concerned Plastic Surgeon.

Pledging to Donate Skin After Death

Any person wanting to pledge to donate one's skin after death can log onto www.skindonation.in and fill up the pledge form online. A Skin Donation Awareness Kit will then be sent to that pledger to make his/her relatives aware about their wish.

> You give but little when you give of your possession. It is when you give of yourself that you truly give.
>
> **Kahlil Gibran**

Bone Donation

Astrid Lobo Gajiwala

INTRODUCTION

The Tata Memorial Hospital (TMH) Tissue Bank was established in 1988, at a time when tissue banks were almost unheard in India, and a few existed in Asia. A pioneer in the field, it is the first tissue bank in India to use radiation for the sterilisation of biological tissues, and in 2004 became India's only Tissue Bank with an ISO 9001:2000 Certified Quality Management System. Currently it banks gamma-irradiated, human amnion, tendons, and bone which are used for its own cancer patients and distributed for use in a wide variety of surgeries in patients across the country.

The banking of tissues begins with the donation of tissues, and a critical person in this process is the hospital's or tissue bank's transplant co-ordinator who is responsible for co-ordinating all matters relating to the retrieval and/or transplantation of tissues. The donation experience begins when the transplant co-ordinator contacts the family of the person who has recently died, usually within a few hours, since the time limit for tissue retrieval is limited. The transplant co-ordinator makes the next-of-kin aware of the possibility of donating tissues. This interaction is conducted with the utmost tact and consideration, as potential donors usually die in unexpected and tragic ways (accidents, heart attacks), and this is an extremely stressful time for the family. Whatever the decision, it is respected, and at no time is there any attempt to coerce the relatives.

While counselling the next-of-kin of a potential donor the transplant co-ordinator is required to answer a number of concerns of the relatives with regard to the eligibility for donation, the procedures for procurement of tissues, the usefulness of the tissues, and monetary considerations. The co-ordinator must also ensure that the donation process is conducted in an ethical manner and that all the pertinent laws are followed.

Frequently Asked Questions

1. What is a Tissue Bank?

A tissue bank is a facility dedicated to the supply of safe, reliable and cost-effective human tissues for transplantation. According to the law, it includes facilities that carry out any activity relating to the recovery, screening, testing, processing, storage and distribution of tissues, but does not include a blood bank.

The tissues are recovered from deceased donors, after brain stem or cardiac death, or living donors who usually donate tissues that are removed during surgical or medical procedures that are conducted for therapeutic purposes. All donated tissues are processed, sterilised and preserved only after appropriate consent of the donor has been obtained, and screening has been performed to rule out infectious diseases and disease of unknown origin.

2. Who can Donate Tissues?

The majority of deceased donors are individuals who were otherwise healthy but who died in accidents or from sudden illness such as a heart attack or stroke.

3. Are there any Age Limits or Medical Conditions that can Prevent one from Being a Donor?

The surgeon or recovery team decides at the time of tissue recovery whether the tissue can be banked. The age limit is different for different tissues.

There are no maximum age criteria for bone if it is to be morsellised, or is not to be used for weight bearing purposes. When large skeletal segments are obtained to provide structural support, the donor should be free of any significant osteoporosis and preferably below 55 years of age.

All donors are screened to rule out infectious diseases, and tissues will only be procured if the donor meets the tissue bank criteria.

4. What does the Donation Process Involve?

Before donation can take place every donor is thoroughly screened to eliminate transmissible disease. This includes physical examination of the donor's body, and asking the family about the donor's medical and social history including questions about HIV/AIDS and high risk behaviour. Blood tests are performed to rule out hepatitis B, hepatitis C and HIV infections. The next-of-kin are asked to sign a consent form for banking the tissues.

The procedure can take anywhere between 1–6 hours depending on the tissues being donated, and must occur within 24 hours of the time of death.

5. Is there a Difference between Tissue and Organ Donation?

Tissue donation is a simpler process than organ donation. Organ (heart, liver, kidney, etc.) donation is possible only after brain stem death, which is defined as the complete cessation of all functions of the brain. Brain stem death is a medical diagnosis which can only be ascertained by a team of certified doctors. In brain stem dead donors, mechanical support (i.e. a ventilator) is required so that the circulation of blood is maintained to continue the viability of the organs for a short period of time after the death of the patient. The donor is usually kept in the intensive care unit. As such the death must occur in a hospital where the necessary support systems are in place. The donor and recipient must be carefully matched according to their blood type, and the transplant must take place within a few hours.

Tissue donation from deceased donors may occur either after brain stem death, or cardiac death (the cessation of the heart). It does not require the donor to be on mechanical support systems and consequently any death is an occasion for potential donation. The time factor too is not as critical as for organ donors.

6. Are there any Problems of Rejection of the Graft as in the Case of Organ Transplants?

Blood-typing is not required for tissue transplants. There are no problems of rejection and anti-rejection drugs are not required to be used in tissue recipients.

7. What Tissues can be Donated?

Deceased donors can donate tissues such as bone, cartilage, ligaments, tendons, fascia lata (the thin covering of the muscles), heart valves, pericardium (the membrane enclosing the heart), veins and skin.

8. Who Procures the Bone?

After the necessary authorization for the donation of tissues has been received from the family or legal representative, the donated tissues are removed in a clean environment by trained professionals in the presence of a registered medical practitioner.

9. Will bone Donation Disfigure the Body of the Donor?

During the donation procedure, the donor's body is treated with the utmost care and respect. Bones are procured in a manner similar to that used during surgery. Clean incisions are used which are neatly sutured after donation.

When bones are retrieved from the limbs, care is taken to reconstruct the limbs to closely approximate their original anatomical configuration, using wooden or bamboo rods that can be incinerated or biodegraded depending on whether the body is finally cremated or buried. Visible areas are left unmarked as far as possible to enable viewing of the body during the funeral.

10. Can Organ Donors also Donate Bone?

Yes, organ donors can also be tissue donors and help many more people. In these multiple donors the organs are recovered first because the time factor is critical. If the eye is being donated this is retrieved after the organs followed by skin and then bone.

11. Are there any Costs Involved in Tissue Donation?

No, there is no charge to the donor's family. The cost of the blood tests is borne by the Tissue Bank.

12. Is there any Payment for Donation?

No, the law makes it illegal to buy and sell human organs and tissues. Tissue donation is similar to any donation. It is inspired by the desire to benefit people in need.

13. How is Bone Used?

Donated bone is used in a number of ways. Generally bone is morsellised (broken into smaller bits) and used to fill cavities in a patient's bone, which may have been caused due to disease or trauma. It can be used for reconstructing skeletal defects or to provide structural support during fracture healing particularly when the bones do not unite on their own. Often it is used to reinforce bone that has been weakened, as in patients with osteoarthritis and those needing total knee or hip replacement. Small segments of bone are used to correct deformities in the spine, for instance in children suffering from tuberculosis, while bone powder is used by dentists to treat defects in the jaw bones.

In patients with cancer, morsellised bone is used to enhance the recipient's bone stock by packing it into the large defects resulting after the removal of tumours. Long bones may be used to replace cancerous bone. Without the bone transplants the limb may have to be amputated, or an expensive imported prosthesis may have to be used which would require repeated revision surgeries.

14. What Happens to the bone After Transplantation?

Once the bone is accepted by the recipient it is slowly converted into new living bone and incorporated into the body as a functional unit. The transplanted bone stimulates the recipient's cells to begin producing new bone, itself acting as a scaffold for new bone formation. New bone cells produced by the recipient creep into this scaffold in a process called 'creeping substitution'. The donated bone is slowly resorbed. This process occurs over many years.

Ethical and Legal Rules

The Transplantation of Human Organs and Tissues Act, 1994 (Act of 1994), and the Transplantation of Human Organs and Tissues Rules, 2014 (Rules of 2014), governing consent and retrieval of tissues from brain stem dead donors shall be followed as applicable.

1. Tissue Donation

1.1. In the case of brain stem death of the potential donor, the transplant co-ordinator of the hospital where the brain death has been declared will determine if Form 10 of the Rules of 2014 certifying brain stem death is signed by all the members of the Board of Medical Experts specified in the form.

1.2. Physicians involved in tissue procurement or transplantation shall not pronounce death nor sign the death certificate of any individual from whom tissue will be collected.

1.3. No removal of tissue will take place when there was an open or presumed objection on the part of the deceased.

1.4. The transplant co-ordinator of the hospital where the brain death has been declared will determine if Form 7 authorising the donation of tissues prior to death is available with the next-of-kin or the donating hospital or the State Organ and Tissue Transplantation Organisation (SOTTO).

1.5. In the absence of Form 7, permission or confirmation of the absence of objection for tissue donation shall be obtained from the next-of-kin. This shall be obtained by the registered medical practitioner of the hospital having the Intensive Care Unit where the brain death has been declared and/or the transplant co-ordinator of the hospital. The next-of-kin of the potential donor must be given appropriate information regarding the importance of the donation for the recipient as well as the option to authorise or decline the donation of tissues.

1.6. Informed consent of the next-of-kin authorising the donation of tissues from the brain stem dead donor must be recorded in Form 8 of the Rules 2014 (Rules 5(4) (b)).

1.7. Even if the potential donor carries a signed donor card, or documents like a driving license wherein the provision for donation of tissues after his/her death is incorporated, or has pledged tissue donation in Form 7 of the Rules, 2014, every effort must be made to contact the next-of-kin and ascertain if the person had subsequently revoked her/his consent.

1.8. In case of brain stem death of a person less than eighteen years of age, Informed Consent shall be obtained in Form 8 of the Rules of 2014 from either of his/her parents or any near relative authorised by the parent (Rules 5 (4) (d)).

1.9. Reluctance to donate on the part of the family must be respected even if the deceased has signed documents to indicate consent (Rules 5 (4) (a)).

1.10. The transplant co-ordinator of the hospital must inform the State Organs and Tissue Transplant Organisation (SOTTO) of the tissues donated (Rules 5 (1) (c)).

2. Medicolegal Cases

2.1. Removal of tissue cannot be effected if it interferes with a forensic examination or autopsy as required by Law. Tissues may be recovered provided the cause of death is not jeopardised (Rules 6 (2)).

2.2. After informed consent has been obtained on Form 8, the transplant co-ordinator of the hospital must seek permission from the local police authorities for the planned retrieval of tissues. A copy of the request and permission received from the police for the retrieval of tissues must be submitted to the designated postmortem doctor of the area (Rules 6 (2)).

2.3. A medical report of the tissues being retrieved must be prepared at the time of retrieval by the retrieving doctor and must be included in the post-mortem notes (Rules 6 (3)).

2.4 In case the tissue donation takes place in a hospital that is not doing post-mortem the hospital must arrange for transportation of the body along with medical records to the designated post-mortem centre (Rules 6 (5)).

3. Monetary Inducement for Donation

3.1. Monetary payment or advantages for the donation shall not be made to the brain-stem dead donor's next of kin or any donor-related party.

3.2. Donors or their family shall not be financially responsible for expenses related to retrieval of tissues, their transportation and pre-servation. The recipient of the tissues, or institution or Government or non-government Organisation or society as decided by the State Government shall bear the expenses and compensate the donor's family for any donation-related expenses (Rules 9).

4. Packaging and Transportation to the Tissue Bank

4.1. All retrieved tissue shall be provided with an accompanying retrieval form including at a minimum, the donor identity, the date, time and place of the procedure, the identity of the person (s) performing the retrieval, the tissue(s) retrieved, the donor and tissue selection information including reports of serological tests.

Copies of the retrieval form, informed consent (Form 8), certificate of brain stem death (Form 10), and no objection from the police in medicolegal cases, shall be dispatched to the Tissue Bank receiving the tissues.

4.2. If an autopsy is performed, the results shall be made available for review by the Tissue Bank.

4.3. Each tissue segment shall be packaged individually as soon as possible after retrieval, in an aseptic manner with at least one moisture barrier, and labelled with the donor and tissue identification, in such manner that traceability of tissues will be achieved.

The retrieved tissue shall be transported at wet ice temperatures (1 to 10°C) or colder. The maximum time that retrieved tissue shall remain at wet ice temperatures prior to either processing or freezing, shall be no longer than 72 hours.

4.4. If samples for microbiological testing are taken, they shall be labelled and dispatched to the tissue bank with the tissues and forms.

Hand Transplant

Vinita Puri

INTRODUCTION

Hand transplantation is a surgical procedure to transplant a hand from one human being to another. The goal of the procedure is to restore function to a person who does not have hands (amputees).

Technically, the surgery is similar to limb replantation but it needs immunotherapy like solid organ transplantation. A hand transplant is different from single organ transplants as it is a composite tissue allotransplantation (CTA), i.e. many body tissues are transplanted together—skin, fat, muscles, tendons, nerves, blood vessels and bone. Each of these tissues have different antigenicity, with skin being the most antigenic organ in the human body.

History

World: The first attempt at hand transplant was in Ecuador in 1964. The first-hand transplant to achieve prolonged success was by a team from Kleinert Institute, USA performed in January, 1999. In Jan 2004, the team from France declared a five-year-old double hand transplant a success. In July 28, 2015, Children's hospital of Philadelphia, performed the first successful hand transplant on a child—a bilateral transplant on an 8-year child and two years later the child is functioning well.

India: On January 13, 2015, at the Kochi-based Amrita Institute, India's first hand transplant was done successfully. The hands of 24-year-old accident victim were transplanted to the 30-year-old man who lost both his hands in a train accident. After that, they have successfully performed two more transplants with the third one being at the above elbow level.

Organisation of the Hand Transplant Team

- Experienced plastic surgeons (experienced in micro surgery and hand surgery)
- Orthopedic surgeons
- Anesthetists
- Transplant immunologists
- Transplant pathologists
- Microbiologists
- Rehabilitation specialists and hand therapists
- Psychiatrists
- Transplant coordinator

The Institutional capability includes

- Dedicated operation theaters which run 24×7
- Transplant ICU and nursing support
- Blood bank (24×7).

Selection of Cases

Recipient Selection Criteria

Patient who accepts and understands the advantages/disadvantages and risks involved in this surgical technique and also understands and accepts the effects of lifelong immune-suppressants.

Patient should ideally have been using prosthetic alternatives before transplantation.

Age: Standard age for transplant is between 18 and 65 years. But this age barrier has been crossed and an 8-year-old child has already received a double hand transplant. So if the patient is healthy and deserves a transplant the patient can be considered.

It is to be remembered that earlier a hand transplant is done, the more the number of years they have to spend taking immune-suppressants. With increase in age, they are more mature to accept the realities of hand transplant and are more compliant with the immunosuppression and rehabilitation protocols.

Single vs. Double Hand Amputees

Risk–benefit ratio—hand transplant vs immuno-suppression.

The risk–benefit ratio in case of *double hand transplants* is more acceptable because prosthetic rehabilitation of double hand amputees does not provide as good a functional recovery as achieved through transplants.

Single hand transplants can be considered in highly motivated patients with a dominant hand amputation and those who are willing to accept the risks of long-term immuno-suppression.

Type of Cases
- Traumatic below the elbow amputation
- Electric burns (assessment of the proximal muscle and nerve function should be done to assess the extent of damage).
- Congenital defects do not qualify for transplant as cortical representation as well as development of muscles/nerves to make tranplanted limbs work may not be there.
- This procedure is also not being considered for individuals whose injury is limited only to fingers.

Psychological Stability

Recipient should be prepared psychologically for daily required immune medications, repeated controls and the possibility of rejection and infective episodes.

Tests
The patient will have to undergo clinical evaluations which will include history and physical examinations, X-ray evaluation, psychosocial evaluation, nerve conduction studies, tissue studies and laboratory studies.

Donor Selection Criteria

Donors will meet the criteria of total and irreversible damage to the brain and the family consents to organ donation. Donors screened according to Indian Organ Donation guidelines.
- Size and blood type are the only donor requirements which are mandatory.
- The gender, skin tone, race and age are more of an individual preference than a mandatory requirement.

Exclusion Criteria
Absolute Contraindications
- Risk of infection transmission
- HIV
- Hepatitis B/C
- Current malignancy
- Limb paralysis
- Peripheral neuropathy
- RA or significant osteoarthritis
- Connective tissue disease

Relative Contraindications
- Viral encephalitis
- Uncontrolled HTN
- Vasculopathy

Counselling of the recipient: Counseling of the recipient and his/her immediate family is done in several sessions independently by the lead surgeons, immunologists and the transplant social worker. The counseling has to be in a non-influential manner.

Negative aspects need to be laid stress upon during counseling sessions rather than promoting the transplant in an unnecessary positive way. The patient has to understand that other than an absent limb they are healthy but use of immune-suppressants could make them feel unhealthy as they would take medicines lifelong and that it would need them to make lifestyle changes and they could have long-term health implications.

Financial aspects of the transplant, need for lifelong immunosuppression and postoperative rehabilitation protocols are stressed upon by the team leaders, therapists and the social workers.

Counselling of Donor Family

Consent will be obtained from the relatives only after explaining the exact nature of retrieval and technique of body restoration.

Prosthetic limb will be available with each team which should be shown to the relatives before donation.

This will be fitted to the donor stump before returning the body to the relatives.

Order of Procurement of Donor Limb

By mutual consensus amongst the organ retrieval circle.

The plastic surgeons can progress with the harvest of limbs under tourniquet control without causing blood loss. Once the limbs are harvested, the other organs can be retrieved.

Aftercare

- After the transplant is over, patient will be kept in the transplant ICU for 2 weeks.
- After that for another 2 weeks in the transplant ward.
- He/she has to stay in the vicinity of the hospital for 1 year.

Immunosuppression Regime

All hand transplant patients need be on immunosuppressive therapy which includes drugs that must be taken every day for the rest of their life. The immunosuppressant drug therapy is similar to the drugs that are taken by kidney transplant patients.

As there is a risk of infection caused by the immunosuppressive drugs the recipients need to make lifestyle changes particularly in the first six months. Some of them are as follows—avoiding people with communicable diseases, avoiding crowds, wearing a mask while outside or in a dusty, crowded place, avoid gardening, etc.

Skin Biopsy Protocol

Skin biopsy is done to assess for the rejection of transplantation instead of serological testing which is done to assess rejection in solid organ transplant. If there is no clinical sign of rejection, then biopsy is taken from proximal half of hand.

Protocol for the skin biopsy is as follows:
- Weekly × 1 month
- 2 weekly × 2–3 months
- Then monthly.

Rehabilitation Protocol

Hand transplant rehabilitation protocol consists of four phases with distinct goals, frequency, and modalities.

- **Pre-operative:** Functional assessments with establishment of goals and expectations.
- **Initial postoperative (postoperative weeks 1–2):** Hand protection, minimization of swelling, education, and discharge.
- **Intermediate (postoperative weeks 2–8):** Therapy aims to prevent and/or decrease scar adhesion, increase tensile strength, flexibility and function, and prevent joint contractures.
- **Late (from 8 weeks forward):** Maximization of function and strength, and transition to routine activities.

Awareness Programs

It is necessary to increase awareness regarding hand transplants amongst lay public and even medical professional. Amputees should be invited for such awareness meetings and encouraged to share their experiences with others. Successful hand transplant patients can also share their life stories of better life after transplantation.

Body Donation

Pravin H Shingare

INTRODUCTION

Donor can donate his organs, tissues or whole body. Body donation is accepted only after cardiac death. Very few organs like eyes, skin, bones, etc. can be used after cardiac death. However, whole body can be used for teaching in medical colleges and also in the colleges of health sciences courses.

HISTORY OF BODY DONATION

First body donation was done by sage Dadhichi, son of sage Chavan and Sukanya. As per Hindu mythology his bones were used to prepare Astra with which Demon Vatrasura was killed. To learn human anatomy, scientists were illegally purchasing dead bodies from grave yard. Italy was first to permit dissection. Then England permitted dissection since 1724. However, British parliament passed Anatomy Act in 1832. India passed Bombay Anatomy Act in 1949.

Bombay Anatomy Act, 1949 Amended up to 30-4-1983

This Act is mainly for supply of unclaimed bodies of deceased person and also covers body donations before death. As per this Act, the said donation is for therapeutic, education, teaching and research purpose only. This Act gives protection from prosecution and no suit will be there against Anatomist. The Act shall not prohibit postmortem. To promote the body donation, the State Government has appointed a "Body Donation Committee" in all Government Medical Colleges headed by Dean. Two social workers and superintendent of the hospital are the members of the said committee.

Body Donation, Why Needed?

There are 50 Medical Colleges in the State of Maharashtra and more than 460 Medical Colleges in India. Total 6500 MBBS seats are there in Maharashtra and more than 63000 MBBS seats in India. To study human anatomy, average one dead body is required for 10 students. Thus 65 dead bodies are required alone in Maharashtra and 630 in India per year. Though more than 1.25 cr. people die in India per year, it is difficult to get sufficient number of dead body donation to learn anatomy for budding doctors (Table 5.1).

Guidelines for Co-ordinators

All co-ordinators and social activists working in this field should have blank forms of body donation. They should know which are the centres where body donation is registered in the nearby area. They should have contact numbers of office bearers of the medical colleges (Anatomy Department) and hospitals where donation is accepted.

Procedure of Body Donation

1. Fill the prescribed form, attach a photograph
2. Submit the form in Anatomy Department or send by post.

Table 5.1: Donation sources

Sr. No	Donor	Consent	Use	Act
1.	Live	His own	Organ (kidney, liver)	THO Act 1994
2.	Brain stem dead (after brain death)	Near relative	Organs (kidney, liver, heart, lung, etc.)	THO Act 1994
3.	Cadaver (after cardiac death)	Near relative	Eye, skin, bone, etc. and whole body	Bombay Anatomy Act 1949

3. Get the registration number and donation card from Anatomy Department
4. Ask donor to inform near relatives about his/her donation.
5. During night hours and on holidays, inform to RMO of the Medical College Hospital about the death of the donor. Bring the body to casualty. RMO will accept it and will kept it in the cold storage. However, next working day, relatives must come to complete the formalities in the Department of Anatomy.

Who Cannot Donate

- Having age less than 18 years
- Patients of HIV, hepatitis, cancer, burn, gangrene
- Cause is unnatural
- If kin is against donation
- If expressed "No Consent" before death

Eminent Body Donors

- Jyoti Basu, Chief Minister of West Bengal
- Shantanurao Kirloskar, Industrialist
- V.D. Karandikar, Marathi Poet
- Madhu Dandawate, Ex-Railway Minister, Govt. of India
- Kamlabai Ajmera, Ex-Minister, Govt of Maharashtra
- Vishwanath Banshetty, Ex-Mayor, Solapur, Municipal Corporation.

Procedure

1. Those who are willing to donate his/her body (after death) should submit a written application to Anatomy Department of any Government/Corporation Medical College alongwith photograph and consent of near relatives.
2. The written application should be in the format which is freely available in Anatomy Department. It can be xeroxed and used by many people. The body donation registration is free.

3. The donor will get a donor card on which instructions are given about the steps to be taken after death by the near relatives.
4. After the death of the donor, relatives should inform to the Medical College where he is registered for donation on the contact number given on the Donor card. Call for a Hearse and shift the body to the Medical College. The College authorities will pay for the hearse charges if within the city as per government rates.
5. Take death certificate from the family doctor (RMP) in prescribed format if home death. The certificate should mention that the death is natural.
6. Medical College authorities will not come with ambulance to collect dead body of donor from his/her home.
7. Handover the dead body to Anatomy department and get a receipt of body.
8. Submit the Doctor's death certificate to the nearby Municipal Corporation Ward Office and bring from them the Death Registration Certificate in the official format.
9. If no pre-registration, still near relative can take decision of donating the body of deceased person. The person in legal possession of dead body can donate for Anatomy Department.
   If relatives demand, then a small piece of dead body can be given to relatives for rituals. However, once donation procedure is complete then the relatives will not have right to see the body or demand for other details. The body donation has to be unconditional. If more number of donors come forward, the quality of teaching, learning will improve and more research can be carried out about structure and function of human body.

Communication and Counselling Skills

Introduction to Counselling in Deceased Organ Donation

Sujata Ashtekar

In India, the Human Organ Transplantation Act, 1994 has paved the way for Deceased Donor Transplantation or cadaver transplantation as it has given recognition to brain death and organ donation. The lives of the patients suffering from end stage organ failure can be saved by transplantation.

Unlike any other surgery, this surgery depends on the availability of a healthy organ. Hence, obtaining consent for organ donation from the close relatives of the brain dead individual is the most important and sensitive aspect.

Counselling is mainly face to face interaction with the person to help him/her cope more effectively with the problem faced. Here, the family is suffering from grief due to loss of loved one and counsellor plays the challenging role of grief counsellor.

He helps them to cope with the feeling of shock, disbelief, sadness, anger, guilt associated with grief. A counsellor working in deceased organ donation further aims to convert the negative feeling due to loss of death into positive sense of helping others and saving many lives by giving them the opportunity to donate organs.

The transplant counsellor also counsels the recipients and their family before and after the transplant surgery. He/she helps them to cope more effectively with their illness, helps them in getting listed for deceased donor transplantation, give them reality orientation about the unplanned nature of the surgery, long waiting period and importance of regular follow-up with the transplant team and the counsellor.

The counselling intervention is necessary to the donor family who is suffering from grief and to the recipient who is suffering from organ failure and to recipient's family.

Abilities of the Counsellor in Deceased Donor Transplant

Every hospital registered for transplantation, needs to appoint a trained transplant counsellor/coordinator who has the basic **knowledge** of medical, social, ethical, legal and religious aspects of transplantation and is capable of answering frequently asked questions related to organ transplant. He/she should have the counselling and communication **skills**. The most important quality of a transplant counsellor is to have the positive **attitude** for organ donation.

Role of the Counsellor in the Process of Approaching the Donor Family for Consent

The donor family can be approached for organ donation by taking conscious steps. In practice, the step may overlap but it makes the process of obtaining the consent a planned and systematic effort and increases the possibility of positive response from the donor family.

Step i: Identification of the Potential Donor

In the first step, the potential donor in ICU is identified. The counsellor should take daily round in ICU to interact and build rapport with the relatives of all the patients. All the relatives whose loved ones are in critical care shall be offered counselling service to cope more effectively with their need and problems.

The counsellor should also interact with the treating physician, intesivists and nursing staff to know the health status of the patients. The diagnosis of the brain dead patients who are likely to be potential donor can be thus facilitated by the counsellor.

The patients with intracranial bleed, head injury, cerebral anoxia or primary cerebral tumors may lead to brain death.

The transplant counsellor organizes for the first set of brain stem death by calling the recognized four doctors from brain death committee [i.e. treating physician, neurologist/ neurosurgeon, specialist, the hospital admini- strator].

The counsellor facilitates the identification of brain death individuals in ICU by organizing training on brain death and organ donation for the sensitization of ICU staff.

He/she maintains file in the ICU for organ donation with the copy of the HOTA-1994, State guidelines, protocol, consent forms, important phone numbers like of brain death committee member. The counsellor also maintains the data of the potential donors identified in the ICU, their eligibility and outcome of the approach to the relatives.

Step ii: Donor Assessment

Once the donor is identified, the counsellor should interact with the intensivist to know that contraindication like malignancy, hypothermia, bacterial and viral infections are ruled out. The doctor can send the basic tests like blood grouping, viral markers, and renal function test. The age of the donor should be between 2 and 65 years as per the Maharashtra State guidelines. The donor up to 70 years are accepted as marginal donors.

In short the donor should be assessed and screened for organ donation.

At this step, the counsellor alerts the retrieval team and the organ procurement or coordinating agency in the city about the possibility of organ donation.

Step iii: Building up Rapport with the Donor Family

The counsellor can interact with the donor family and build up rapport with them. The treating physician can formally introduce the counsellor to the family.

In this step the counsellor can do family assessment in terms of the no. of close relatives being present. As per the law only close relatives can give consent for organ donation and the term close relative is defined as spouse, father, mother, brother, sister, son, daughter. The counsellor needs to motivate close relative to sign the consent form.

The coordinator also assesses who is/are the decision maker/makers in the family. If the extended family members are more open and interactive, their help can be taken to approach and motivate the close relatives.

The coordinator can take case history; know from where the family belongs. The socioeconomic background of the family and their religious orientation can also be assessed.

The family is continuously informed about the health status of their loved one. Slowly, they are prepared that the prognosis of their patient is grave.

Step iv: Declaring Death to the Relatives by the Treating Physician

After the first set of brain stem death, tests are done including **apnea** test, the treating physician can declare brain death to the family. This should be done in the presence of counsellor who is going to make request for organ donation. The terms like "life-support" and "patient" should be avoided. The death has to be clearly informed to the family without any ambiguity.

Decoupling

The counsellor should not make request to the family about organ donation when the family is told about death. Some time should be given to the family to acknowledge death before raising topic of organ donation. Declaration of death and the request for organ donation should be decoupled. In practice there has to be two separate interviews with some time gap to declare death and to make request for organ donation.

Observe the Stages of Grief

When the family is told about the brain death of their loved one they go through various stages of grieving process like denial, anger, bargaining, and depression and finally they will accept the death. These stages may overlap.

Denial: In **denial** stage they may just refuse the death of their loved one. The statements like "His heart is still beating" or "This can't be true" are made to refuse the death.

Anger: There can be **anger** expressed on themselves or on the hospital staff. This has to be taken as their coping mechanism and the counsellor should never take it personally. He/she can be silent and still available and helpful to them.

Bargaining: In the stage of bargaining, the family makes statements like "Don't worry about the cost and do whatever to save our loved one" or "Can we shift him to the bigger hospital for the best treatment." Thus family tries to negotiate with the counsellor for the result which shows they have not yet accepted the death.

The counsellor should never make request when the family is in the stage of anger, denial or bargaining.

The family may express their sadness and anguish by crying in the stage of depression. Slowly, they may accept the death after going through various emotions and make statements like "what next?" or they would like to inform death to other relatives.

The counsellor should interact with them to help them cope with the loss and cope effectively. The counsellor should provide the family privacy, water, phone facility and assist them. The nursing and the security staff should be told about how to deal with the relatives of the brain dead individual

especially about when and how family should be allowed inside the ICU.

Step v: Making Request for Organ Donation

The request for organ donation can be made when the family accepts the death of their loved one. The counselor should confirm that at least one set of brain stem death including apnea has confirmed the brain death of the donor. The coordinator should make a request when most of the close relatives and decision makers are around. The best timing for making request is when the counsellor feels the family is in the stage where they can listen to the topic of organ donation.

Dos while Approaching the Family

The approach should be made by the counsellor in the presence of intensivist and senior nurse taking care of the patient. The team of doctor, nurse and the counsellor sit face to face with the family to make a request is considered to be the best approach.

- The family should be provided with the sitting arrangement and the privacy. A staff room in ICU can be used for this purpose.
- All the queries of the family related to brain death should be answered repeatedly.
- The family should be informed about the utility of brain death by sharing that they are in a unique situation where they have the opportunity to help others in their grief as the organs can be taken only from the brain dead individual.
- The counsellor can help them to empathize with the recipient by telling them how the organ donation is the only ray of hope for those who are dying with the end stage organ failure.
- The counsellor can boost the donor image by saying that the donor must have been the helpful person in his life and whether he would have liked to help others by donating organs.
- The donor family can be motivated to donate by sharing that something positive can come from death and many lives can be saved.

- The counsellor can overcome myth related to organ donation by sharing the facts like:
  - It is legal to donate organs. The organs are distributed as per the priority criteria given by the govt. guidelines and are not sold to the rich.
  - The body is given back to the relatives after the organs are retrieved in the OT.
  - There will not be disfigurement of the body but there would be cut and sutures like any other major surgery.
  - All the religions in India support organ donation.
- The counsellor should avoid giving false promises to the donor family with regards to the timing of giving back the body or the waiving of hospital bills.
  It should be clearly told to the family around 5 to 6 hrs. would be required to complete the procedure of organ donation and no money transactions are allowed in return of organ donation.
- Make open ended statements while making a request like "In spite of making the best efforts we were not able to save your loved one but now you can think to help others and save many lives. You all can discuss and let us know."

Counselling Skills

Listening skills: The counsellor should listen to the verbal and nonverbal messages of the family. Listening is the most important quality of the counsellor which helps to convey the message that he/ she is concerned about their problem.

Genuineness: The counsellor should be at herself and spontaneous. When the strong emotions are expressed, the counsellor may feel uneasy and the best technique is to be silent or allow the family to grieve its own be available to them.

Be non-judgmental: The counsellor should not be biased depending on the religion, educational and financial status of the family. Every family should be approached for organ donation and should be given opportunity to donate.

Express acceptance: Be available and accessible to the family irrespective of their response. Express warmth and support. It is important to show the same support to the family even if they refuse to donate organs.

Step vi: Taking Consent from the Family

After making the request allow the family some time to consider organ donation.

If the family responds positively then take written consent on Form no. 6 and 7 and take signature of the close relative. If donor is a minor take consent of the parents on form no. 9 along with Form 6 and 7.

Be with the family till the body is handed over to them.

Send a letter to the donor family appreciating their act and how it has saved others without revealing the identity of the recipient.

The counsellor can do long-term follow-up by sending death anniversary cards, etc.

Thus, by taking conscious and systematic steps the counselling of the donor family and the request for organ donation can be made. The refusals by the families should be evaluated, analyzed and documented by the counsellor which would help her to be better in her next approach and would serve as important research data.

Recipient Counselling

The deceased donor transplant is a major surgical activity and the recipient has to come for the surgery without any notice whenever the donor is available. The recipients also need help to cope more effectively with their illness. Hence, the **pre-transplant counselling** where the recipient is helped to get prepared for the surgery is essential.

The physician of the recipient or the patient suffering form the end stage organ failure may refer the patient to counseller.

The counsellor interacts with the recipient face to face to inform him that the deceased donor transplant is the established therapy available to him/her if there is no possibility of getting the organ from close relative. The counsellor gives reality orientation to the recipient about the deceased donor programme and also motivates the recipient to get listed in the city waiting list.

The counsellor helps the recipient on the following aspects:

- The recipient is helped with the procedures of getting registered on the city waiting list.
- The recipient needs to be financially prepared the details of the cost of surgery and immunosuppressant are discussed and family of the recipient is helped to prepare for the same.
- The recipient is informed about the unplanned nature of the deceased donor transplantation and he is regularly counselled that he may be called for the surgery any time without prior notice.
- The recipient is given reality orientation about the long waiting period before they get the organ and continuously informed about their priority on the waiting list.
- The recipient is also informed about how the organ are distributed on the basis of priority criteria like age, status of illness, etc.
- The recipient is advised to come for regular medical follow-up and inform about the change in contact numbers, if any, to the counsellor immediately.
- The counsellor can facilitate the support group in the hospital of all the listed patients which helps them to feel that they are not the only ones suffering and helps them to cope effectively with their illness.

Conclusion: Counselling is the backbone of the deceased donor transplantation programme.

Donor Family Counselling

Bhavana Shah

INTRODUCTION

Every organ donation is different, clear communication with the family or next-of-kin is essential to helping them understand brain death and their options for organ donation. The transplant coordinator coordinates a network of medical, para-medical and non-medical personnel. They are key to create a positive outcome and help the families of brain dead individuals. Their role in counselling the families for organ donation is instrumental in making the programme successful.

Transplant coordinator may have to play different roles such as, grief counsellor, motivator, advocate, educator and change agent.

It is unfortunate that many families have never discussed or even thought about organ donation until a tragedy happens. Families will be asked about the wishes of their dead relative. If these wishes are not known, the family will need to make the decision. Families need information and answers to their questions before being able to process information about organ or tissue donation.

It is also critical to have an understanding of family dynamics and identification of the legal next-of-kin as that person may be different than the person making health care decisions. Transplant coordinator can start building rapport with the family to understand the following:
- Who are the decision maker in the family?
- Socioeconomic status
- Religious things, etc.

Counselling Skills of Transplant Coordinator
- Be a good listener—listen to their verbal and non-verbal messages
- Be genuine
- Be non-judgmental
- Express acceptance

Questions Essential to the Decision-making Process
- What happened to their loved one? What is the nature of the injury to the brain and the patient's prognosis?
- What is being done to care for their loved one or to save his or her life?
- Family members need to be able to see their loved one.
- Family members need to have detailed information and time to understand "brain death" concepts before any mention of donation.
- Explanations and information often need to be given more than one time to family members.

As a Grief Counsellor, it is also important to understand what time we are giving offer the opportunity for donation or requesting for donation it should be an appropriate time, because there are situations that may complicate the grieving of family members and family go through different stages of grief like

Denial: The request for organ donation may come as a shock for many relatives.

Family can deny when you put request for Organ Donation initially.

Anger: It is difficult situation for the family and they may be aggressive in the following situations:

- Sudden death
- The death of a child
- Perception that death may have been prevented
- Lack of support
- Lack of opportunity to spend time with their relative.

Bargaining: Family can bargain like:

- Some time they may request give one organ to our family member who are suffering from organ failure.
- Can a family get lifetime medical facilities for free of cost, etc.

Negotiation: They always try to negotiate in billing.

Acceptance: Means only after the family understands their loved one is dead.

One important point for Transplant Coordinator: Never make a request when the family is in the stage of anger/denial/bargaining.

Support for donor families will help in their grief recovery

- Accurate information regarding the patient's treatment and likely outcome
- Empathy and understanding from all staff
- Information about organ donation
- The chance to ask questions
- Private times with their relative and a time to say "goodbye"
- Consideration of spiritual needs.

What Happens Once Family Accepts to Donate?

After acceptance, usually family will have plenty of questions.

What Does the Donation Operation Involve?

The donation operation is conducted with the same care as any other operation, and the person's body is always treated with respect and dignity. This operation is performed by highly skilled surgeons and health professionals. Specialist doctors and their teams may be called in from other hospitals to perform the operation.

Similar to other operations, a surgical incision will be made in order to retrieve the organs, and this incision will then be closed and covered with a dressing. Depending on which organs and tissues are being donated, the operation can take from 3 to 8 hours to complete.

What Happens after the Operation?

Following the operation, the donated organs will be transported from the operating theatre to the hospitals where transplantation will occur. If the family would like to see their loved one after the operation, this can be arranged.

Will the Person Look Different?

When a person dies, it is usual for them to appear pale and for their skin to feel cool, as blood and oxygen are no longer circulating around the body. However, the donation operation does not result in any other significant changes to the person's appearance. The surgical incision made during the operation will be closed and covered as in any other operation and will not be visible beneath the person's clothes.

Will Funeral Arrangements be Affected?

Organ donation will not affect the arrangements required for funerals. The body can be viewed properly. If a Coroner's investigation is required, this may delay funeral arrangements.

When is a Coroner's Investigation Required?

Some deaths, such as deaths from unnatural causes or where the cause of death is unknown, are required by law to be investigated by the state or territory Coroner. In these circumstances, a coronial autopsy may be required. The hospital staff will discuss this with the family if it arises.

Can the Family Change their Minds about their Donation Decision?

Yes. The family can change their minds about donation at any point up to the time when the patient is taken to the operating room.

What are the Religious Opinions about Donation?

All religions support organ donation. If a family has any questions they would like to discuss, the hospital staff can provide them with additional information, and assist them in contacting their religious leader.

Will the Person's Family be Expected to pay for the Cost of Donation?

No. There is no financial cost to the family after death has been formally certified.

Which Organs and Tissues will be Donated?

The doctors will discuss with the family which organs and tissues may be possible to donate. This will depend on the person's age, medical history, and the circumstances of their death. The family will be asked to confirm which organs and tissues they agree to be donated. They will be asked to sign a consent form detailing this information.

Does the Person's Family have a Say in who Receives the Organs and Tissues?

No. The allocation of organs and tissues is determined by transplant teams in accordance with ZTCC protocols. The organ allocation depends upon scientific criteria and waiting list so that outcome of the donation is optimum.

Will the Person's Organs Definitely be Transplanted?

If the family supports donation, everything possible will be done to make sure those wishes are fulfilled. At the time of retrieval or donation, sometimes organs are found unfit for transplantation. The hospital staff will discuss this with the family if it arises.

Is Transplantation Always Successful?

Are all hospitals recognised for its successful transplants and its long-term survival of recipients. As with any operation, there are some risks associated with transplantation surgery, however, the majority of recipients benefit greatly from their transplants and are able to lead full and active lives as a result.

Will the Family Receive Information about the Patients who have Benefited from the Donation?

Indian law restricts identifying information being shared between donor and recipient families. However, the donation staff will provide ongoing information about which organs and tissues were transplanted, and the progress of the recipients. Donor families and transplant recipients can write anonymous letters to each other through the state or territory donation agency (e.g. ZTCC).

It is important to show the same support to the family even if they say "No" and respect their decision. Organ donation does not take away the pain of death. However, many donor families have said that the transplant was the only positive thing to come from the death of their relative.

Counselling Process

Rekha Barot

INTRODUCTION

Cadaver donation process is defined as the set of actions and procedures that can turn a potential donor to an effective donor. Counselling the donor family is an important part of donation process. Counselling process in Cadaver Donation is one of the toughest jobs in the world.

Major difficulty faced is convincing grief-stricken relatives of a brain-dead person to give organs of their dear ones and this has to be done within a limited period of time.

Three Key Stages for Approaching the Families of Potential Organ Donors

1. Preparation and planning of the family approach
2. Discussing brain stem death
3. Request for organ donation

1. Preparation and Planning of the Family Approach

The preparation and planning is very essential for presenting the possibility of donation at the right time and in the right way. The way you talk to the family, the way you explain the diagnosis, the donation process and the assistance you give to the family at that time, will direct the family for donation or not.

Prior to initiating a family approach, the consultant, the transplant coordinator and the intensivist should meet in private to discuss and outline how the request process should proceed. If a meeting is not possible, they should participate in the planning process by telephone. This is a key stage in the process and gives opportunity to the transplant coordinator to discuss clinical issues, assessment of the patient's donation potential and the implications of organ retrieval with the treating doctors.

The transplant coordinator should check the medical records to know the name and background of the potential donor; the cause of death and how it has happened. It is important to identify the characteristics of the family in advance, since one family is different from another and there are aggressive people, docile people and inquiring people.

It is important to arrange for a room with privacy for counselling the family. The presence of a professional from the institution who accompanied the case is important to give credibility to the process and support the interviewer.

Sometimes the participation of people who have no kinship with the potential donor or family, who are not considered legal representative for the decision regarding the donation, may interfere, disrupt and influence the legal representative person in decision making. Therefore, for the interview to be performed, it is important to consider the degree of relationship of the person who will be interviewed and their involvement and proximity to the potential donor. It is better to identify next of the kin and decision maker in the family and talk to them. In India it is usually a male member. To improve the interview, it is also important to identify the person with greater discretion and understanding of the facts. Sometimes it is better to talk to them in group as there may be dissenting members in the family who are against organ donation—on the spot judgment often required.

Important points to be considered during counselling

- Extensive use of counselling and communication techniques such as listening, observation, exploration, ventilation, informing, logical discussions, etc.
- To make eye contact with relatives
- Be yourself and be spontaneous
- Be genuine, empathetic and non-judgmental
- To act without bias regarding religion and financial status
- To show compassion for those in grief
- Relatives to be treated with respect
- To make the family feel comfortable (get water and food if desirable)
- To listen well to what the family wants to tell and ask
- To make efforts to overcome myths
- To explain everything repeatedly.

2. Discussing Brain Stem Death

In general, an open communication style atmosphere allows the family members to express their fears and desires. The ultimate goal in discussing death with the family of the deceased person is to optimize their comfort and alleviate any fears.

Let the family know you are ready to talk to them whenever they are ready for it. Forcing information will usually result in anger, distrust and emotional distance from others. Waiting until someone is ready to handle the situation will allow for better communication.

Grieving families have feelings of sadness, confusion, anger and fear. It is essential to react in an appropriate way to these emotional reactions and to connect with whatever the relatives want to tell or ask.

As a routine, a treating physician or intensivist would be expected to lead the breaking bad news conversation before making the transition to the transplant coordinator, who will lead on the discussion.

The way of reporting death to the family and the moment at which the topic of organ donation is broached exerts great influence on the outcome of the donation procedure. Disappointment, anger or frustration with regard to the procedure should be prevented by handling the situation as carefully as possible.

It is important to understand that each person and family is different. Given that different cultures have varying beliefs about death, there is no single right way to discuss death.

To start the conversation it is always good to ask the family what happened and show compassion for their loss. At the same time build rapport with the family. It is important to have clarity while explaining brain death to the relatives. It should be explained in simple language avoiding medical jargon. Relatives expect calmness and attentiveness in conversation.

It is vital to spend time ensuring that relatives have full understanding of brain death before discussing organ donation. The key is to give the family as much time as they need and to use language that leaves no room for any doubt whatsoever that brain stem death is death—not its likelihood, not its inevitability but death itself. Utilising diagrams and scans are the ways in which a family can be supported through such uncertainties. These interactions need to be done courteously and credibility needs to be established over a period of time when the relatives are going through extreme grief.

Decoupling: The process of separating the talks related to death and organ donation is called decoupling.

Families who have not yet come to terms with the inevitability of their loss will not be in a position to consider donation. Indeed it would be unfair to expect them to do so at this point. It is essential that clinical staff explicitly consider whether family members are ready to consider donation, and that if there is any doubt suggest a 'time out' that allows the family to reflect upon the clinical reality of the situation and to come to terms with it. This is sometimes referred to 'decoupling'. Clinicians should not underestimate how much time families need to come to terms with the fact that their loved one has died, especially if it involves a child or young adult.

However, there are families—frequently those who have already accepted the situation before the formal discussion—who may be ready to move onto the possibility of donation within the same meeting.

3. Request for Organ Donation

The most important but also the most difficult and sensitive step in the process. Prior to discussion of donation, prevent unplanned or premature mentions of donation by hospital care team. Make sure that family demonstrates understanding of patient's prognosis and brain death before any mention of donation.

The moment to ask for donation can be difficult to pick especially in a situation like in road traffic accident cases where time is very important. You cannot wait for too long after first declaration of brain death as most cadavers are unstable will generally collapse. But, on the other hand, you do not want to approach the family at the wrong time. Therefore, the first thing to do is to observe the state of the family. A request for organ donation should be avoided in stages of denial, anger or bargaining.

In the next step, it is good to repeat the explanation of brain death and ensure that they have understood it properly.

At all times, the language regarding donation should be positive, emphasising the potential benefits for recipients, their families and society in general. The known benefits to donor families in the longer term should also be mentioned, whilst the use of negative or apologetic language—such as "I'm sorry to

bring this up, but..." or "you understand that it is hospital policy that we always ask..." should be avoided.

As eye donation has become quite common in India, it is logical to start with a request for eyes. Subsequently you can proceed with explaining about organ donation and make a request of other organs.

Some sentences which can be helpful in conversation

- Donation is an opportunity to help others
- It is the only hope for many patients
- Death can bring something positive in this way
- Organ donation has the ability to save and transform up to eight other people's lives, starting tonight

Always communicate gently and offer options without any pressure. Give honest and accurate information to family members.

Do not give false promises regarding time of giving back the body after organ retrieval. Relatives should be given enough time to decide about organ donation and should not be pressurized to decide quickly.

Some frequently asked questions during conversation

- Can't he or she come back to life after brain death?
- Will the face/body be disfigured?
- Our relative carried a donor card but we object, what will happen?
- Will donation delay the funeral /cremation?
- When will the donation take place?
- Will our decision make a difference?
- Will we hear about the recipients?

Though back up arguments are extensively used to convince the family for organ donation, yet, the right to self-determination of the attendants is always accepted.

If the family agrees, then consent is taken from near relatives.

Importance of Communication Skills and Organ Donation

Sucheta H Desai

INTRODUCTION

Communication *per se* simply means imparting or exchange of knowledge. To be in contact and to maintain the contact is possible by means of communication only. The communication can be in different ways. The method of communication and the frequency can vary as per the requirement in the situation. Man is a social animal, although he may deny wanting any support from anyone, but somewhere in the corner of his heart, support is usually welcome. It can be from a family member, a friend, a colleague, a teacher, or it can be just the presence of a person with good intentions for him.

Communication can be by

Talking: It is important to gauge the background of the person, to be able to converse accordingly; adopt a soothing way of talking; give the required information; explain in simple language; clear a misunderstanding/misconception, and whatever other clarifications that are required. During the conversation body language is important, in fact, it plays a very big role. Body language of both matters, i.e. speaker and listener. Ours can make us reach out to the person/s (the donor family) to be able to confide, inquire and to empathise. The attitude with which they react to the news, the expression, the tone of their speech, all give us a reading of the type of acceptance or rejection our communication is having on

them. Composure and cordiality are compulsory requirements.

Listening: Be a good listener. Have short timely inputs so they know that you are in the flow of the dialogue. Eye contact, posture and expression (body language) also matter a lot.

Touch: A touch on the hand, a pat on the shoulder or back, a hug, a ruffle on the head, etc. are examples of small gestures which can go a long way to build and maintain a rapport.

Visual· Picture memory is very strong. Explanations through pictures, animations, videos, movies. These can overcome a language barrier.

Acting: Enacting characters, role plays, plays, skits, pantomines, etc. A type of communication, which is carrying a message can be impressionable. When conveyed through these means, again, a language barrier is overcome.

Audio: Soothing talks and music, motivational discourses, chantings, relaxing techniques. They are also very effective forms of communication and help in creating a relaxing environment.

Appliances: Radio, telephones, TV, computers, appliances, etc. These gadgets make distances vanish and communication very easy. Some of the above communication methods come into play in public awareness programmes.

It has been observed that, at times of stress, or during crucial decision taking times, more so in unexpected and sudden situations, the need to share and exchange opinions or advice becomes an important necessity. The decision maker may be one but sharing of the pros and cons makes all the difference. Considering consent for organ donation after declaration of brain death and requesting for organ donation is such an event.

In Case of a Potential Organ Donation

On the declaration of brain death all the above situations come into the picture!... the world suddenly comes to a standstill, it's a sudden jolt, a halt or the world just falls apart! It is a state of shock, an impossible occurrence! First the news was imparted that the condition of the patient is bad, the options of treatment are discussed and explained, no improvement, the prognosis is poor, damaged brain cells do not recover, the patient's brain has stopped working now! The brain is dead. Brain death is also death. In brain death only there is the option to donate the organs, i.e. the organs which require a blood supply, the solid organs. There is no bank for these organs.

What all understand and know about as death is cardiac death. Herein, heart stops, blood flow stops, body cold, breathing stops, monitor shows straight line. In this way of death the person is not eligible to be an organ donor.

Donation of eyes, skin, other tissues can be done. They are preserved in the respective banks. One can also do a full body donation.

The first reactions of the family on the declaration of brain death...

- How can this happen? To him? To us? His family?
- It was just headaches on and off! The patient came in walking! The surgery went well!
- The patient was walking, talking and dancing and enjoying himself at the party just one day ago.
- He was not injured, just thrown off the bike, his friend who was driving the bike was bleeding!
- He only had slight headache and giddiness since some time, no illness!

- He had gone to the bank, he just fell flat on the ground!
- She was cooking, suddenly complained of a headache and just sat down, taken to hospital, now this!
- Brain haemorrhage in a child?

This is a state of shock, disbelief, inability to accept the situation, the mind is in a state of total denial. These situations are usually sudden events, hence unbelievable for the family most of the time. In such a situation it is important "to be there", and "to be with them". Thus, an apt support, the unsaid communication, and just being around helps a lot. At the time of declaration of brain stem death, which is done by the treating physician, it is necessary to provide for a private sitting area or a room for the donor family. The explanation of the meaning of brain stem death, is explained by the primary physician, ideally in the presence of the transplant coordinator.

Information regarding the patient's condition was always being shared by the doctors in the ICU with the family members. Only after the declaration of brain death, the option of organ donation is now communicated to the family of the potential organ donor. Give time to accept death, in the initial stages of grief, do not request for organ donation. In this time of grief try to support, have some tissues, water, tea available for the distraught family.

After declaration of brain death

- The coordinator's role to request for organ donation comes in here. Introduce yourself, explain your role after brain death declaration. Inquire what is their under-standing of the treating consultant doctor's declaration and explanation. Explain further in simple layman's language.
- Call all family members together, identify the decision maker. Explain the special option available to the patient. To be an organ donor. To be a life giver, vision giver! Only in this way of death (brain death) is one given this option of donating organs, as the situation is that—the patient is dead

but the organs are still alive, only due to the machine support.

The family may still ask "Are you 100% sure! No hope at all? May not recover? Coma, people recover after some months also?

Body is warm! Chest is moving in breath! Monitor is perfect, heart-BP all is fine! How is it death?

In these situations education doesn't count, initially only emotions rule!

At this time one has to keep them cool and be able to answer and explain all their queries. After their doubts and fears are cleared, they may decide to donate.

Effective communication is needed to make them understand this situation. Explain that brain death is a way of death, he is not in a coma. The patient is dead but the organs are alive, hence can be transplanted into someone who is already wait listed for one at ZTCC. The positive angle for the donor and family is that, in such a tragedy also they can turn it into a gift of life for more than one, the donor remains alive in another body. Giving life is the highest form of donation. Hence supported by all religions.

We also need to explain the need for the donation. The number of patients wait listed and since how many years. The registering organisation, ZTCC, which has a transparent scoring system and distribution method.

We have to avoid giving promises which may be impossible or difficult to keep. Ideally a donation should be unconditional. They also should be told about the cooperation of the whole ICU staff. The requirement for any procedure on the donor which is required to test functions of the donor organs is always communicated and explained regularly to the family.

The doubts after consent are different

• How will you decide who will receive the organs? Can we give it to someone we know? Do you charge for the organs?
• How many hours will the whole process take? Will the body be disfigured?
• Can we know the recipient's names?

• Will the donor family get some type of support, specially financial help?

Communication has to be maintained in many areas for a positive outcome. Teamwork always yields good result:

• Maintain a good rapport with the ICU nurses, doctors. They are always with the patient. Communication with them is very important.
• Connect with the potential donor family in a general way.
• Counselling for organ donation is only after the declaration of brain death is made by the Primary treating physician.
• Communicate to them about the full procedures happening to the potential donor.
• The need to contact ZTCC, the laboratory for tests, the operating teams, OT, other tests to gauge the organ functions, crossmatching.
• Contacting the probable recipients.
• Explain the approximate timeframe required for all this and for result of the matching.
• The time required in case of a medicolegal case wherein a police NOC for organ donation is required and post-mortem also.
• Easy communication with the ICU nurses, doctors, technicians, billing department and of course the donor family goes a long way in making the whole donation process smooth and stress free for all.
• Try to be there when the body is taken to the OT. Leave a contact number for communication. Coordinate for peaceful release of the dead body from the hospital in an ambulance/hearse. Arrange for the morgue if required.
• The donor family should feel happy and content with their decision to donate and satisfied by the answers to the questions coming to their minds... just by good communication.

Communication and cordiality continues even when...

• The family is in a total "denial state" and refuses to donate.
• The family is motivated and eager to donate but disappointed as the organs are not fit for transplant.

- The organ donation process is completed.
- Even after the body is taken home by the family for completing the last rites and rituals. Do make a call to inquire if all went well.
- The family can be contacted for awareness programmes. Contact for felicitation. Give support in any way that is possible

Many a times, the biggest communication problem is,

"We Do not listen to understand; We listen to reply"

So, communicate, give a proper hearing, and there will be proper answers.

Recipient and Family Counselling and Coordination with Different Organisations

Anirudha K Kulkarni

It is a well-understood fact that human health is still of prime importance for all of us. All people should remain "Niramay" is our ancient prayer. And in achieving this goal, everyone of us has to take help from various sections of the society.

In adverse conditions, we come across different type of people suffering from deadly diseases and they are trying to get rid of them. They have to put up a great fight while surviving. In certain cases, like kidney, liver, heart and organ failure, transplant of organs become necessary. Such surgeries are certainly trying and very complicated. That is for both sides the surgeon and the patient. The patient is a suffering soul and his relative, in a confused state of mind. While surgeon being naturally busy and engrossed in his expert work is unable to communicate with the patient or the relatives at length.

Counselling the word itself mean it includes convincing the individual to reach positive apex point to serve society with social sense. The word counselling has a strong meaning in the world of Organ donation and transplantation.

In India, the enactment of transplantation of Human Organs Act, 1994 (amended up to 2011) started a new era in the field of organ transplantation in general, and role of transplant coordinator for counselling and liasoning with various authorities for compliance, in particular.

Transplant Coordinator

He/she may be a healthcare professional—doctor, nurse, allied health science graduate, or a medical social worker—who coordinates activities related to organ donation and **transplantation**. Transplant coordinators are either donor coordinators or recipient coordinators.

Transplantation of Human Organs (Amendment) Act in 2011 has laid down a set of prerequisites for hospitals to get registered as transplant centres. Appointing a transplant coordinator is one of the prerequisites. The Act defines a **"Transplant Coordinator"** as a person appointed by the hospital for coordinating all matters relating to removal or transplantation of human organs or tissues or both and for assisting the authority for removal of human organs.

It starts when a patient is identified as brain dead in intensive care unit (ICU). In the routine visits of concerned visiting doctors and intensive care unit in-charge, a constructive decision is to be taken in such cases, they certainly continue to give updates about the status of the patients to their relatives.

The medical parameters of the patient show the brain steam death. The doctors help the relatives to accept the death of their loved ones. At this juncture there is dire need of a sympathetic, informative sharer, a bridge between the doctors and the relatives of the patients.

The coordinator is one such person. They are involved in supporting the relatives. They explain the status of the patient to the relatives in very simple language. It is just possible that the relatives find it difficult to understand the medical terminologies. They may have queries about the status, myths and misconceptions about the type of death. They may have some superstitions also. Here the coordinator has to explain to the relatives all these doubts and clarify them. At this point the coordinator introduces the thought of organ donation.

The coordinator keeps a watch on the family background. He also cares for their emotions, mental and social condition in such critical moments. He is also trying to guess the response of the family in favour of organ donation. The coordinator should be sympathetic to the relatives who are suffering from such a loss. The act of organ donation has ability to comfort family members. They can realize the fact that, the loss of their loved one, may help to save/improve the lives of others. The support from friends, religious and cultural beliefs also help donor families. Most of the donor families agreed to donated organs because they felt that, it was the only positive outcome from their loss.

The discussion moves ahead, the relatives of on asking numbers of questions to the coordinator. He should keep calm of his mind and help the relatives. His goal is to prepare them mentally for organ donation. Here the relatives may have questions regarding myths, second opinion, billing, allocation of organs handing over the donor and further unexpected complications.

The coordinator has to clear all these doubts and queries. It shows the commitment towards the donor family and support to the relatives. It may change from negative to positive decision.

The coordinator himself should have positive approach towards organ donation. His communication skill is equally important. His knowledge in this field as well as various religious and cultural aspects must be sound and accurate even his body language should contribute to the ultimate cause.

Coordination with Different Organizations During Cadaver Organ Donation

Coordinator is in charge of all legal, technical, scientific and administrative issues relating to organ donation and transplant. They generally oversee the entire process of diagnosis and deeming a corpse fit for donation and must also faithfully enforce rules.

Related to legislation for the whole process fall under their authority. It is almost a twenty to twenty-four hours journey for the coordinator while performing cadaver Organ Donation.

He is to see a number of authorities in this connection. It is certainly a skillful job to achieve coordination of all related agencies.

He must visit the local police station and also that police station where the first FIR was done. He has to contact HLA (give long form) test centers which is nominated by allocation authority.

Allocation—organ distribution center (Zonal Transplantation Coordination Committee) is to be contacted for donor information and allocation. He should also make arrangements for the operation theater for respective donor hospital. Retrieval teams for kidney, liver heart, skin, and cornea should be ready. He has to coordinate with the respective nephrologist and liver physician.

After the retrieval once donor is shifted to ICU it is must to call police for inquest Panchanama. Where police authority will complete the formality and hospital will handover the body for post-mortem. Police accompany with the donor and relatives for PM. Nearest civil hospital is the appropriate place for post-mortem.

Arrangement for ambulance service along with RTO permission for green corridor becomes necessary. The security side of donor hospital must not be overlooked.

The coordinator should not lose sight of the practical side, i.e. billing department. Hospital can give the only relaxation to the relatives. Hospital can waive off the bill from first set of brain death confirmation (Apnea). At the same time ICU arrangements must be ready. The hospital management should be constantly contacted and coordinator should keep them informed about the current status.

Another important aspect is to coordinate with brain steam death committee. He has to look after the recipient and the donor relatives also.

In fact, his/her work is tough and complex which requires dedication concentration and knowledge. This is an unbiased professional work, he has to facilitate the dialogue between the doctor and the patient.

As he is expected to furnish the donor family with adequate information so he is also expected to share with the recipient family. At this point he should also remember to inform the blood banks and blood donors. The pharmacy staff should also be adequately informed about such transplant so that the medical store is well prepared to provide the required medicines and drugs for operation theater and ICU.

Sometimes media also comes in the picture. It becomes necessary to keep them informed with facts. The coordinator has thus to weave a close network of medical, paramedical and non-medical personal.

The success of organ donation and transplant programme depend on smooth and trained coordination. It is up to the coordinator to create a positive atmosphere. It is really a complex job.

One very important ethical point need to be mentioned herein that, there are many laws pertaining to organ donation. But looking at the present state, it can be seen that those laws need to be amended and modified. Moreover, there is a growing human tendency in every walk of life to find loopholes in the law. So the laws in this connection should be foolproof.

Above all there is the conscience of the coordinator because, like teaching this is also a noble profession. It is our conscience that can very well put a check on the violation of laws.

So organ transplant coordinator should have a holistic approach towards his work. This philanthropic work can give a human being a new lease of life.

Grief Counselling Skills

Arati Gokhale

INTRODUCTION

Transplant coordinators play a crucial role in counselling for organ donation and coordination and these are the key factors for the success of the deceased organ donation programme. Most people need honest and accurate information regarding the status of a patient. People communicate their fears and concerns in many ways: Crying, yelling, ignoring others, seeking information from others, and writing letters. These feelings of sadness, confusion, anger, and fear are all acceptable. It is essential to react in an appropriate way to these emotional reactions and to connect with whatever the relatives want to tell or ask. It is important to understand that each person and family is different. Given that different cultures have varying beliefs about death, there is no single right way to discuss death. In general, an open communication style atmosphere allows the family members to express their fears and desires. The ultimate goal in discussing death with the family of a deceased person is to optimize their comfort and alleviate any fears. Let the family know you are ready to talk to them whenever they are ready for it. Forcing information will usually result in anger, distrust, and emotional distance from others. Waiting until someone is ready to handle the situation will allow for better communication.

For the purpose of organ donation, counselling the family is something that has to be done within a short period of time. However, the relatives will most likely be in a state of grief and denial. Good understanding of stages of grief will help effective counselling.

Different Stages of Grief

Grieving is a normal response to a loss. The grieving process varies from person to person in terms of the order in which one deals with the stages of grief, as well as the time it takes to go through the stages of grief. Spouses of the deceased, children, parents, siblings, and other family members will all experience grief. Psychologists and researchers have outlined various models or phases of grief. In 1969, Elisabeth Kubler-Ross identified five linear stages of grief that most people are now familiar with:

- Denial
- Anger
- Bargaining
- Depression
- Acceptance.

Kubler-Ross originally developed this model to illustrate the process of grief associated with death, but she eventually adapted the model to account for any type of grief. In the study done by Kubler-Ross, she has noted that there are five stages of grief and certain stages may be repeated over and over again throughout life.

Denial: **"This can't be happening to me."**

Denial is a stage where people try to believe that the event is not happening to them or their family.

They refuse to accept facts, information, reality, etc. relating to the situation concerned. One may feel numb, or in a state of shock. Denial is a protective emotion when a life event is too overwhelming to deal with all at once. It's a defence mechanism and perfectly natural.

Anger: It is expressed as why did this happen to me and how should be blamed.

Anger is a stage in which you understand the demise but are very upset and angry that it has happened to your friend or family member. One of the best ways of dealing with bursts of anger is to exercise or participate in another type of physical activity. Talking with family and friends, other people who have gone through the same process, and the hospital staff may also be helpful.

Bargaining: It is expressed as do this and in return I will do that.

I will climb the seven hills of Tirupati by foot or will make a big donation to a poor home and so on ..."

Questioning God, asking "Why us?" and "What did we do to deserve this?" are common questions in this stage. It is normal for the family of the deceased person to make bargains with themselves or God, in the hope that this will make the event to be undone. Guilt is taken as the family feels personally responsible by some action for the death to happen. People tell themselves or God that they promise not to do something they previously did (such as arguing with family members), or to start doing some thing they have not done (such as going to church regularly) in exchange for their recovery. It is important to remember that there is nothing that you, your family member, or friend did that contributed to the death. It is no one's fault.

Depression: Depression and Sadness is Common

This is a stage in which the death can no longer be denied and those involved may feel a profound sense of sadness. This is normal. It can be accompanied by physical changes such as trouble sleeping or excessive sleeping, changes in appetite, difficulty with concentrating on simple daily activities, or feeling a constant fear that something will happen to someone else in the family. Depression may manifest as lack of sleep, lack of appetite or inability to do normal daily activities.

Acceptance: "I'm at Peace with what is Going to Happen/has Happened."

Acceptance is a stage in life. You have made an adjustment to the loss. This does not mean that you will never feel the loss, but you have accepted the death and are at a point where it has been incorporated as part of your other emotions. Usually families find that they are better able to manage their lives overall upon reaching this stage. Going through the grieving process is the best way to cope with a death. By giving yourself and your family permission to grieve, you will be able to cope. The way of reporting the death to the family and the moment at which the topic of organ donation is broached exerts great influence on the experience of the donation procedure. Disappointment, anger or frustration with regard to the procedure should be prevented by handling the situation as carefully as possible. It is important, for example, to have clarity when explaining brain death and how the doctor or nurse reacts to the relatives' emotional outburst. Relatives respect calmness in the conversation, attentiveness from doctors and nurses, and they need to be treated with respect. Also, they prefer no medical jargon to be used. These interactions need to always be done courteously and credibility needs to be established over a period of time when the relatives are going through extreme grief. Unless the family comes forward to donate the organs of their loved ones, it is better to raise the issue of organ donation after declaration of death after the initial period of grief and shock starts sinking in. Relatives generally indicate that they often get too little time to realize that their beloved one has passed away. They appreciate it if they are not pressurized to decide quickly about the donation request. When they get the opportunity to say goodbye in their own manner, they will lookback on the donation procedure with more satisfaction.

Grief Related with Organ Donation Process

It is very much important when one can ask for organ donation, as mentioned above donor family members are suffering from stages of grief, so first counsellor should be able to identify who is the decision maker and that person should be approached The moment to ask for donation can be difficult in many MLC cases as process may be tiring for relatives, where time is the essence. You cannot wait too long after the first declaration of brain death as most cadavers are unstable and will generally collapse. But on the other hand, you don't want to approach the family at the wrong time. Therefore, the first thing to do is to observe the state of the family. The counsellor should avoid making a request for organ donation when the family is in the stage of anger, denial or bargaining. It is best to be with the family right from the time a serious patient is admitted to the intensive care unit and counsel all patients' family irrespective of brain death. In short, daily ICU round with intensivists is much more needed and you as counsellor finished one step of rapport establishment. Such an ICU counsellor is the best person to ask for consent for organ donation and will understand the family

better. To start the conversation, it is always good to ask the family what happened and show compassion for their loss. In the next step it is good to repeat the explanation of brain death, to ensure that the family has understood it and create a rapport with them at the same time. Because eye donation has become quite common in India, it is logical to start with a request for the eyes. Subsequently you can proceed with explaining about organ donation and make the request for all organs and tissues. You should always communicate gently and offer options without any pressure. If the family agrees you can take the family consent on Form no. 8 and 10. If family members give consent for organ donation, counsellor has many more things to do like arranging recipient management, crossmatching, informing police for NOC and panchanama, OT bookings informing ZTCC/allocating organisations, hospital bills, etc.

While doing this all, counsellor should not neglect donor family members and follow some important facts:

- Be a good listener (*listen to their verbal and non-verbal messages*)
- Be genuine
- Be non-judgmental
- Express acceptance
- Be respectful
- Become comfortable with silence.

"It is important to show the same support to the family even if they say "No" and respect their decision".

Protocol for Organ Donation

ROTTO-SOTTO (West Maharashtra), Astrid Lobo Gajiwala, Sujata Ashtekar, Urmila Mahajan

ORGAN AND TISSUE DONATION IN BRAIN STEM DEAD (BSD) DONORS

Step 1. Identification of a potential donor

The ICU in-charge and doctors are responsible for identifying a potential BSD donor in the ICU. However, the Transplant Coordinator has to facilitate the process by:

A. Taking daily ICU rounds and collecting data of patients on ventilators;

B. Developing a rapport with the families of all ICU patients, reviewing the donor's case history, noting the close relatives present and identifying the decision makers;

C. Communicating with ICU doctors and treating physician/unit Head about the call for apnoea if brain stem reflexes are absent;

D. Coordinating with the designated administrator for the first set of brain stem death tests including apnoea.

Step 2. Screening for HIV, active infection and malignancy

Check the patient's file for recent blood reports and any history of active infection and malignancy. Inform the ICU in-charge in case any of these diseases are present.

Step 3. Conducting the first set of brain stem death tests including apnoea

The authorised committee of doctors for declaration of brain stem death will do the tests to certify brain stem death.

A. If the test is positive, note the time for the 2nd apnoea test. In the case of adult donors, there must be a minimum gap of 6 hrs. and in the case of paediatric donors, a minimum of 12 hours.

B. If the test is negative, keep a record of the results.

Step 4. Informing the family about brain stem death

The family is informed about brain stem death of their loved one by the ICU in-charge or treating physician. The transplant coordinator is present when the death is declared.

Step 5. Approaching the close relatives for organ and tissue donation

A. Conduct a face-to-face interaction with the relatives of the potential donor in a room or as private a place as possible.

B. Ask open-ended questions.

C. Give the relatives time to make a decision.

Step 6. The donation process

A. If the relatives agree to organ and/or tissue donation, inform the ICU in charge and the authorised person in the hospital.

B. Inform the coordinating agency [e.g. ZTCC] providing details as per the donor information protocol.

C. Check that Form No. 10 for certification of brain stem death has been completed with all the four signatures of the authorised brain stem death committee.

D. Take the written consent of the relatives for organ and/or tissue donation, on Form No. 8 after the second apnoea test. Take signatures of as many of the close relatives present, as possible.

Step 7. Medicolegal case

A. After the first apnoea test and consent of the relative, inform the police station nearest to the hospital where the case is registered about the possibility of a potential donor.

B. Give a written request to the police to conduct an inquest and to give an NOC for organ/tissue retrieval after the second set of brain stem death tests have been conducted.

C. The post-mortem is done after the organ and/or tissue retrieval.

Step 8. Organ/tissue retrieval

A. The donor is shifted to the operation theatre for organ/tissue retrieval. After the procedure has been completed, the body is respectfully handed over to the relatives.

B. If it is a medicolegal case, after the organ and/or tissue retrieval, the body is sent for post-mortem. The coordinator accompanies the family to the post-mortem centre.

Note: In practice the above steps may overlap.

Step 9. Coordination with city coordinating agency (e.g. ZTCC)

Coordination with the city coordinating agency [e.g. ZTCC] takes place throughout the donation process:

A. Ask the coordinating agency for the list of recipients in the donor hospitals.

B. Send the donor's blood for crossmatching to the laboratory recommended by the coordinating agency.

C. Communicate with the recipient hospitals and coordinate with their recipient teams for retrieval time.

D. Inform the traffic police in the nearest police station about the timing of transport of the organs and the hospitals involved, in order to arrange for a "green corridor".

Public Awareness, Motivation and Ethics

Importance of Public Awareness and Sensitisation in Organ Donation

Sujata Ashtekar

RATIONALE

Human organ transplantation is the achievement of modern medical science in which it is possible to replace a damaged or failed organ by a healthy organ through a surgical procedure. This established therapy is the only ray of hope for patients suffering from end stage organ failure.

Unlike any other surgery, in transplantation, a healthy organ is required to proceed. Use of artificial organs is not feasible, established or accessible yet and will not be an affordable option to many of our end stage organ failure patients. Xeno-transplantation means taking an organ from animals for transplantation. This is also not a possible option due to ethical issues and immune-incompatibility. Science also fears that the diseases which are confined to animals will get transmitted to the human race. Hence, the only possible and ethical way to get an organ to save a human life is from another human being.

It is possible to take an organ like one kidney, a part of the liver, a part of the pancreas or a part of the intestine from healthy living persons because the donor can continue to live a normal life after donation. But, organs like the heart or lungs cannot be taken from a living person but only from brain dead donors. Kidney is the most commonly transplanted organ from a living person to a needy patient. In the past, commercialisation of organs like kidneys [kidney bazaar] led to exploitation of

the poor and needy. To ban commercial dealings of organs and to have a regulation on retrieval, removal and storage of human organs, Human Organ Transplantation Act was passed in India in 1994. The act clearly specified that a living person can donate an organ to his/her near relative; and the term 'near relative' is defined as the spouse, father, mother, brother, sister, son or daughter. The 2011 amendment has included grandparents and grandchildren as well. The living person can also donate to a patient out of love and affection. In these cases permission from State Authorisation Committee is mandatory before performing the transplant.

The act on one hand has put a limitation on taking an organ from living donors and on the other hand has paved the way for organ donation in India by giving recognition to brain death. The act has allowed retrieving all the organs and tissues for transplantation and save many lives if the consent is obtained by the near relatives of the brain dead individual.

In countries like Spain there is an **OPT OUT** system where every citizen is an organ donor unless he expresses that he/she does not want to donate. Thus, here a citizen opts out from organ donation.

In India, we have gone for the **OPT IN** system of consent for organ donation, where a citizen above 18 years of age can pledge to donate his organs after death for therapeutic purposes. If no such pledge is made, the near relatives of the deceased can give consent for organ donation. A citizen has to opt in for organ donation. Hence, awareness for organ donation is important so that more and more people opt in for organ donation.

Why is there a Need to Create Awareness and Sensitize Public on Organ Donation?

Huge gap between demand and supply of organs/shortage of organs

In spite of having many transplant hospitals and the best transplant experts in our country, it is estimated that 5,00,000 people die every year in India while awaiting an organ.

In Mumbai on any given day approximately 3000 patients are waiting for a kidney, 200 for a liver, and 40 for a heart. [The numbers are smaller for other organs when compared to kidney, as patients awaiting livers or hearts die earlier, whereas kidney patients have an option for dialysis]. As per the statistics of ZTCC, Mumbai, from 1997 to April 2017 there have been 320 brain dead donors who donated solid organs and 569 kidneys, 214 livers and 58 hearts have been transplanted. Organ donation rate in India is 0.5 per 10 lakh population compared to 30 per 10 lakh population in the western world.

Due to shortage of organs more living-related kidney transplants are done in India. Where as in Western countries there is tremendous guilt in taking an organ from a healthy relative and around 90% kidneys used for transplantation is from deceased donations. In India, Surgeons have to opt for living-related liver transplants due to shortage of cadaver livers.

Promoting deceased donor transplant programme is the only ethical and practical option for any long-term successful transplant programme. Hence, need for public motivation becomes crucial.

Lack of awareness about organ donation

When the Act was passed in 1994, the people in Mumbai to some extent knew about eye donation but were not aware about the donations of organs like liver, heart, etc. The word kidney was associated with the infamous history of organ selling.

With the continuous efforts by the concerned NGOs, Government Departments, and due to media coverage over the years, by 2017 the coordinators working in the hospitals of Mumbai observe that the people are aware of organ donation. There are many voluntary donations where relatives themselves come forward for donations after death of their loved ones. National Organ and Tissue Transplant Organisation [NOTTO] has received around 12 lakh pledges as per the online report of 'More to Give' Campaign. [Nov, 27, 2016, 12:32 IST, sites.ndtv.com/moretogive/] Though the awareness is rising in the recent few years, these figures are miniscule when compared to our population and a lot needs to be achieved.

Lack of awareness about brain death

Brain dead donor looks like any other comatose patient on a hospital bed and his/her heart is still beating. It is difficult for the family to accept death if they have not heard of brain death before. People need to be made aware that death can also be caused due to irreversible damage to brain stem and brain stem death is death. It is different from coma, and it is definitely not mercy killing.

Religious beliefs

The idea of organ donation is linked to death and funerals and needs to be discussed with the relatives of the deceased. Family members want to perform last rites and rituals as per their religious beliefs. They fear whether their religion allows organ donation or not. They also fear whether they will be born without that organ in the next birth if they decide to donate. The transplant experts and NGOS working in the field have contacted various religious leaders and have taken their support to promote organ donation.

In India all religions support organ donation and consider it as a noble cause.

Myths

There are common myths associated with organ donation which need to be debunked to increase organ donation.

Myth: Organ donation will lead to disfigurement.

Truth: No, it does not disfigure the body. There will be a stitched surgical wound like any other surgery performed on a living patient.

Myth: Body is not handed over to the family for last rites.

Truth: Unlike body donation, in organ donation, the body is handed over to the relatives for last rites.

Myth: Organs are given only to the rich.

Truth: Organs are distributed in a transparent manner as per the priority criteria laid down by the State and are allocated by the government formed coordinating agencies. All transplant hospitals are members of these agencies. Money or economic status is not the criteria for distribution.

Myth: The donor family will be given financial compensation.

Truth: No payment is made to the donor family as it is illegal to do so. It is a noble decision taken to save lives without expecting any financial returns.

Why is there a Need to Sensitise Medical or Para-medical Professionals?

Organ donation in a hospital is a team effort. Patients and their relatives who come to a hospital for treatment look towards every doctor or staff member as the hospital representative. It is important that all those who are working in the hospital are aware about organ donation and speak positively about it. Hospital is a place where every pledge can be converted into organ donation. Brain death or death can occur in any hospital, hence all the medical professionals even though they are not the members of a transplant hospital should be aware about organ donation and be sensitised towards it.

Efforts have been made to include the concept of organ donation and brain death in the medical and nursing curriculum, regular CMEs are organised for general practitioners, nursing staff, ICU doctors and the staff.

The pamphlets and information on organ donation should be easily available in every hospital. Posters on organ donation can be displayed at waiting areas.

The awareness among professionals is the first step which will lead to optimisation of approaching the family of every potential donor irrespective of their religion, caste, creed, economic and social status and educational qualification.

Aims of the Awareness Campaign

- To educate professionals and general public about the importance of organ donation.
- To provide information about organ donation pertaining to what, when, where and why.
- To debunk myths in the society related to organ donation.
- To bring about a positive attitude towards organ donation in the society.

Target Groups for Awareness

Every citizen is required to be made aware about organ donation. It is important to focus on medical and para-medical professionals as well as police personnel, forensic experts as they play an important role in the process. A transplant co-ordinator should regularly plan awareness activities within the hospital he/she is appointed at and at the nearby police stations too. A transplant coordinator has to plan and interact on a micro as well as macro level. Awareness can be done at individual, group, community and mass level. Social media can be used effectively to spread the message.

Individual level: This involves directly providing information on organ donation to individuals through face-to-face interaction or telephonically or by providing pamphlets. A helpline should be available on which individuals can contact to make enquiries. This method may not help to reach a large number of people but gives quality information to those who are interested. A donor card, information pamphlet and organ donation form is given to each individual.

Group level: This involves interacting with various social groups existing in the community. Power point presentations, awareness talks or interactive sessions, quizzes on the topic can be organised. For example, Mahila Mandals, youth groups, senior citizen groups, Rotary and Lions club, groups of corporate employees, school and college students, NSS students, religious groups, etc.

Community level: The message can be spread through various community gatherings and events like Ganesh festival, *Pandharpurvari*, Marathons, etc. and at places like railway stations, bus stops, malls, temples, churches, etc. Awareness can be spread by displaying posters, putting stalls, forming human chain, organising marches, performing street plays and flash mobs.

Mass level: The social message is spread through print and electronic media. In print media, coverage of all the donations made is promoted so that more people get inspired. Articles are written by experts in the magazines.

In electronic media, interviews of the experts on organ donation or chat shows on the issue can be telecasted regularly; coverage of donations done is encouraged. Radio can also be an important medium to promote the cause.

There is need of a massive National Campaign through print and electronic media which can make organ donation reach the masses.

An Organ Donation Promoter should target all the levels. The individual organ donation activists, hospitals, concerned Government Departments and NGOs should build alliances and collectively work towards promoting organ donation and turn it into a social movement.

Motivation for Organ Donation

Meera Suresh

"Please Do Not Take Your Organs to Heaven—God Knows We Need Them Here"

What does this line mean to you? Does it make you think about making a decision to donate your organs when you leave this world?

The requirement for organs is increasing day by day—there is a big gap between demand and supply. Where do you go when you need a kidney, a liver, a heart, an eye or some skin? There are countless questions such as, "How do we get Organs?", and "Who donates them?" That we help you find answers to, so that you may, in turn, enlighten others across the country.

Many lives can be saved if vital organs such as the heart, liver, kidneys, lungs and pancreas are available for transplant. Unfortunately, in India, the availability of organs is abysmally low and thousands of patients on the waiting list die each year.

While the law permits live donor transplants amongst blood relatives, it does little to make available organs to those who have no suitable blood relatives, to receive donations from. Many families not only lose their near and dear ones waiting for the organs, but also face financial crises in their efforts to keep the patient alive and run the family thereafter. This situation leaves the family physically, emotionally, and economically drained.

Deceased (cadaver) organ donation, (in case of brain stem death) if encouraged, will therefore both save lives and ensure the welfare of the families. In case of normal deaths, skin and eyes can be donated within 6 hours of death to give sight and save burn patients. The retrieval teams arrive to harvest the tissues within an hour of being summoned. There is neither bleeding nor any disfigurement, and the donor's body is bandaged and wrapped properly and handed over to the family with due respect, and in full dignity.

Myths and misunderstandings such as, *"if we donate eyes, we shall be born blind in our next birth"* and *"skin donation will disfigure the body"* are plenty. The truth is that, burns patients heal in half the time required normally because of the donated skin. One brain stem dead donor can save up to 9 lives. Organ donation is absolutely legal. Besides, each and every religion supports organ donation and considers it a very noble cause.

People have to be motivated to donate and not think about organ donation only when your loved one needs an organ. If you can take an organ when you need it, you can also donate them when your need is completed in life.

Motivate—spread the word: There are 3000+ patients awaiting kidneys, 250+ for livers and 20 for hearts only in the city of Mumbai.

We can all do the best for spreading the word about organ donation by informing our family, friends, relatives, colleagues, residential building members, social groups, NGOs, senior citizen groups, and social organizations, and spreading the word in our Social Media circles like on Facebook, WhatsApp, Twitter, etc.

Formal education about organ donation may begun right from 9th and 10th school grades, and continued into college. Teaching and non-teaching staff as well as NSS and NCC groups can be involved and asked to arrange awareness programs.

Every organisation, government, non-government, corporates, banks, under their CSR Projects, in fact, anyone and everyone has to be educated. Each one of us can be Ambassadors of Organ Donation.

Giving your organs after death is not just about making a donation; it is about making a difference. Do not think that organ donation is giving up a part of you to keep a stranger alive. It is actually a total stranger giving up a large part of them to just keep a part of you alive. In the end, one must realize that each one of us is born with the unique ability to change someone's life. We must not waste it.

The tremendous efforts in spreading awareness among people all over India, and some states have really caught up with this drive. Inter- and intra-state organ transplants have now become possible with the **"Green Corridors"** which help in transporting the retrieved organ within minutes and hours and conserving vital time lost in transportation.

For example, the organs retrieved from a cadaver are kept in a solution and frozen in an icebox. To maintain the quality of the organ to be transplanted in a recipient's body, which will be beneficial to the patient, the timing is most important.

The maximum time permissible from the time of the retrieval to transplanting the organ in the patient is only 4 hours in case of heart, 8 hours in case of liver, 12 hours in case of pancreas and 20 hours in case of kidney. Beyond this duration, the quality of organs starts deteriorating and they will not be fit for transplant. Therefore, if organs are received from outside Mumbai, they are airlifted first and then the Traffic Police/Police are alerted well in advance to control traffic and clear the entire route from the Airport to the hospital. Hence, it takes only minutes instead of hours, which is very vital as the quality of the organ should not deteriorate before it reaches the recipient. A cadaver donation requires precise coordination between Transplant Co-coordinators and retrieval teams, pathology teams, recipient hospitals, operation theatres, the donor family, and the recipient families.

We believe that you, as responsible citizens, can help us in several ways, mainly by organizing awareness camps in your area, societies, offices, social groups, religious groups or during community events. We hereby seek your active participation in supporting this noble cause.

Developing of Educational Tools, Mass Mobilization and Campaigning

Sandip Bhurke

INTRODUCTION

Public opinion on various subjects is very fluid. It can change as per further inputs and propaganda from various government and nongovernment agencies. Goodness in the heart of the public needs to be awakened and channelised. Organ donation and specifically eye donation usually has special good feel response from the public.

Planning an Awareness Drive

A public awareness health talk on organ donation needs to be streamlined and conducted in the following steps:
1. Arranging series/program
2. Speaker requirements
3. Interactive talk with internet media involvement
4. After interactive talk ends

Choice and Character Composition of Audience and its Organizers

Time Required

Minimum time required to convey message of organ donation and concept of brain stem death: The terminology of "lecture" should be changed to "organ donation health awareness interactive talk".

Organ donation requires the audience to understand the concept of heart beating brain stem death deceased donor in whom the organs are still alive. This concept requires approximately minimum 8 to 12 minutes to be understood by the audience.

Location: Usually the concept that death can be a reality despite a beating heart causes amazement in the minds of the audience. Hence, constantly flowing or walking crowd like railway platforms, religious gatherings and festivals and places like temples, masjids, gurudwaras, churches, etc. should never be taken up for organ donation health talks. In these places the audience attention span is hardly 5 to 10 seconds. Also, the audience will take away the pamphlets and literature and use it as coverings for prasad, etc.

Prior arrangements: The main impetus for the health talk comes from dedicated organizers who would arrange for covered seating area, air ventilation and audiovisual aids. The organizers would send out prior intimation (pamphlets, SMS, WhatsApp, emails). The Health talk may be part of a larger program of the institution or organizers program, e.g. Republic Day, prominent person felicitation day, etc.

Always keep the health awareness talk in the middle of two other lectures. At first initial lecture the audience is still arriving or settling down and the dignitaries and trustees may not have arrived still. Awareness talk at the end of series may not be successful as the audience starts walking out to refreshments, food or exit. Do not distribute organ donation pamphlets at the reception table at the beginning of the talk. Keep distribution of pamphlets and donor cards at the end as a special publicity event.

The talk: Breakup the available time slot into 5 parts:

a. Introduction and felicitation of dignitaries, trustees, speaker and ZTCC coordinator. Lighting of ceremonial lamp if in the agenda.

b. Powerpoint health awareness interactive talk with 3 special slides.
  i. Decapitation
  ii. Headless but alive chicken
  iii. Anencephaly baby

c. Large size ceremonial donor card with local organization logo already printed on it. Distribution to dignitaries and trustees with prior intimation and permission.

d. Distribution of donor cards and pamphlets set to audience with photograph each time

e. Vote of thanks

Adjust as Per Audience Character and Discipline

Army and police will take maximum registrations for donor cards.

College students will take maximum photographs and spread the message widely on social media like facebook and WhatsApp.

Give official announcement at start of meeting that at the end of the program audience members should take photograph standing with speaker while accepting donor card and pamphlets set in their own mobile. The audience members are requested to send these photographs from their own mobile to their own WhatsApp and facebook. Simultaneously official photographer takes official photographs on official camera for website of trustee organizers and ZTCC.

Requirements for the Speaker

- Should have letter from ROTTO/SOTTO/ZTCC for authority to take the talk
- Should come down from the stage and walk in between the audience for maximum impact
- Should keep stethoscope over shoulders to impress upon audience medical information.
- Should keep smile on face

- Keep separate person to change the presentation slides.
- Keep presentation slides as question and answer format.
- Keep presentation in multiple and local languages (e.g. shivaji 01 font for Hindi and Marathi. This is simple to type and easy to install in control panel of computer).
- Use cordless hands free collar mike, microphone so that both hands are free. This is connected wirelessly to speaker amplifier.
- Send by email the presentation and regional language font 2 days prior to organizers. No virus spread as by pendrive.

After the Talk Ends

- First ask for fund raising for ZTCC/ROTTO/SOTTO and distribute the request for donation letter.
- Then request the dignitaries to come on stage.
- Large A4 size ceremonial donor cards with organization logo already printed are distributed to trustees and dignitaries. Before start of program each dignitary and trustee must be informed of the small ending program of accepting ceremonial donor cards. Rarely some person may not want to accept donor cards.
- Thereafter take photograph of each trustee accepting ceremonial donor card. Again take group photo with trustees and dignitaries holding ceremonial donor cards.
- Request all audience members to come one by one on stage and to take photograph standing with speaker while accepting donor card and pamphlet set in their own mobile. Simultaneously official photographer takes official photograph on official camera for website of trustee organizers and ZTCC.
- The audience members are requested to send these photographs from their own mobile to their own WhatsApp and facebook. This spreads the message worldwide.
- The trustees and organizers are requested to send back a thank you letter to ZTCC/ROTTO/SOTTO for record keeping for Charity Commissioner's office with feedback of programs done during the year.

Ethics in Transplant

Joseph Thomas M

INTRODUCTION

Solid organ transplantation can be considered as one of the most significant achievements of modern medical science. This was made possible by the advances in surgical techniques, anaesthetic drugs and procedures and modern antibiotics. This was coupled with a better understanding of the immunological mechanisms and refined methods to modify the rejection of the transplanted organs. Transplantation of kidney, liver and heart has become and established replacement therapy. Lung, pancreas and intestinal transplantation followed with good success rates. Currently uterus and hand has also been successfully transplanted, though in a smaller scale. Unfortunately this success of modern medicine also saw the emergence of many ethical, moral, legal and social issues which were intertwined with each other. The public outcry in India against the rampant kidney trade involving unscrupulous dealings for money resulted in the Transplantation of Human Organ Act in 1994, the Parliament of India. This was subsequently adopted by the various states who framed the Rules for the proper implementation of the provisions of the Act. The main objectives of the Act was to promote cadaver transplantation and prevent the commercialisation of organ donation. There was a provision for unrelated live donor transplantation for altruistic reasons with the approval of the Authorisation Committee. This well-intended provision has been much maligned provision and used in an unethical way with exchange of money.

A paired organ like kidney or a part of an organ like liver could be removed for transplantation from an appropriate live donor. But the removal of the whole liver or heart mandates that the patient is "dead". There were attempts to remove kidney, liver or heart immediately after the heart stopped beating and the person is officially declared dead. This was often not possible due to logistic reasons and the organ thus harvested may be less than ideal. Corneas were regularly harvested after the death of a person as it remains viable for a longer time. This necessitated bringing in the concept of brain death and redefine death. Brain death is a state of irreversible damage to brain after which in a varying period of 12–36 hours will lead to cardiac arrest and death. This usually followed severe head injury, massive stroke, brain tumours and complications of neurosurgical procedures. These brain dead patients are usually diagnosed in intensive care units which will be equipped to maintain them on artificial ventilation and a beating heart. It will be possible to conduct a planned operative procedure for multi-organ harvesting before the patient is finally declared dead. Many countries including India has accepted "brain death" as a legal concept and has enacted special laws on organ transplantation. THOA 1994 in India was an important step that legalised the concept of brain death making harvesting from brain dead donors feasible and has since then largely replaced non-beating heart donation or the true cadaver donation.

The concept of brain death has been accepted as a legal provision which has made organ donation from brain dead person possible. But there are many ethical issues faced by the brain stem organ donation program and are summarised below:

1. Concept of Brain Death

This is a proven medical concept of death where there is irreversible loss of function of brain and brain stem. This concept was difficult for an ordinary person to accept that death has happened in a person with a beating heart. But the public awareness has increased with more and more people accepting the concept of brain death. The religious beliefs also play an important role in accepting brain death.

2. Brain Death Linked with Organ Donation

THOA has linked brain death with organ donation. This means that when somebody accepts organ donation after the brain death, then the culmination of events with organ harvesting is easy to accept. But if one is not willing for organ donation after brain death, then it is not possible to stop life support as per the existing laws. This can be construed as a form of coercion for organ donation. It would have been prudent to delink brain death from organ donation. There is also a misconception among the public that death is hastened by declaring brain death so that the organs could be harvested.

3. Whom to Talk of Relatives

It is important that the potential donor family is approached with a request to consider their brain dead near one as a potential donor of organs. This is often the starting point of a brain dead donation. At the time of grief and sorrow, it needs trained counsellors to approach the family. The family should be able to address their doubts and questions and make an informed choice. It is important to have the medical person who was the primary care physician to be involved in this initial process. At the same time it is important that the members of the transplant team are not involved at this stage as it be misconstrued as a vested interest hastening death for a faster organ donation. It is necessary that there is a process in place to provide the necessary personal and social support for the relatives in their grieving process. The words should be used with care. For example, donation is a dignified word than harvesting.

4. Consenting Issues

There are two type of consenting in brain death donation.

The *Informed consent* given by the close family after the declaration of brain death. At this time of personal grief it requires a motivated person to talk to and comfort the relatives and request permission to consider the possibility of organ donation. In an emotionally charged situation doctors are often reluctant to suggest organ donation. This is the most important role that a transplant coordinator can fit into and motivate the family for organ donation. It is absolutely important to honour the wishes of the dear ones even if they are not willing for donation. It is heartening to note that many of the dear ones would like to donate the organ from their near ones so that it will continue to live in another needy person's body. It is also important to take only organs for which the relatives have given permission.

Presumed consent: The doctor can use the organs from a brain dead person if he has no reason to believe that the person has not expressed his wishes to not donate the organs after his death. This gives an opt out option for the person when he was alive and in its absence organs can be used. Many of the European countries have given the opt out option.

5. Relatives Willing but Unsuitable Donor

The awareness among the public about brain dead donation has significantly improved.

More and more people are coming forward giving permission to use the organs of their dear ones once the futility of treatment is explained to them. But it is not uncommon to find that the organs are not suitable due to medical reasons. It is important that the Counsellors explain these and appreciate their willingness for organ donation. It will go a long way in improving the awareness of organ donation.

6. Costing Issues in the ICU

The declaration of futility of treatment and the possibility of brain death usually happens in an intensive care set up. The donor will be on mechanical ventilation with all supportive care. Once they are declared brain dead it is important to maintain them like any other patient till the organs are harvested in a planned way. This means that the intensive care bed will be occupied till harvesting. The cost of maintaining the patient in a fit condition for donation often works out to be a significant amount. The bed and monitoring facilities also will not be available for another sick patient who may need it to sustain life. Major attitudinal changes are needed from all the involved personnel to achieve the optimum result. The relatives often want everything to be over fast so that they can carry on with the ceremonies associated with death. But it takes time from declaration of brain death to the time when the body is finally handed over to the family. The family is often concerned about the escalating cost in the ICU. It is natural that they expect the waiver of the charges by the hospital. But is it ethical to waive off the whole amount as it can amount to a form of undue inducement for donation? Is it right to think that the hospitals waive off the money for a noble reason? It is also possible that the hospitals may not be too keen to be part of an active brain dead donation program due to these factors. As most of the ICUs where the potential brain dead donors are maintained are in the private sector there is a potential for skewed allocation of the organ favouring the private hospital. This is more so as one of the paired organ goes for the harvesting hospital.

7. Incentives for the Donor Family

The basic concept of organ donation is that there should not be any monetary transaction in the process of transplantation. There has been many discussions on the pros and cons of giving incentives to the donor family for their selfless action. It can be in the form of waiver of the hospital bills after the declaration of brain death to facilitating final rites by transporting the dead body or payments for funeral rites. While this is a noble gesture for a family in their time of grief that some of their immediate financial concerns are met, it should not be form of undue inducement. The socioeconomic strata of the potential donor family is so varying in the Indian context that it is impossible to form any guidelines across the country in this regard. It will be more beneficial if a local body can decide upon this and decide on the local needs.

It will be a good thought to give some recognition to the family of the organ donor. It can be in the form of a public appreciation of their selfless deed. The other thoughts like educational support, preference in jobs or preference in the organ waiting list in the untoward situation of one of the family members needing an organ later are good. But the implementation needs much to be thought off.

8. Shifting to Another Centre

The earlier policy of harvesting in a recognised transplant centre necessitated the shifting of the patient. The relatives were often not happy with this arrangement as they wanted to complete the formalities as soon as possible. There was also the possibility of soft incentives that were offered to preferentially shift the patient to a particular hospital. The provision of non-transplant organ retrieval centre has improved this situation to a large extent.

9. Handling of Bodies and Helping in Completing Formalities

The earlier days of brain dead donation saw many obstacles for the completion of the formalities. This was often necessitated by many of the patients being medicolegal problems many legal formalities had to be completed before handing the body to the relatives. But the proactive steps by the government in making the procedure simpler has significantly reduced the time taken to complete the formalities. The provision of completing the medicolegal formalities in the operation theatre including post-mortem examination after the completion of the organ harvesting is a welcome move in this direction.

10. Allocation of Organs

The allocation of the harvested organs was always a debatable point as there are not enough organs to meet the needs of all the persons who need it. It is important that the financial or educational status, race or influence in society should not influence organ allocation. It is common to see the relatives requesting that the harvested organ of their relative be given to one in their own family who needs it. The present system of having a centralised list and allocation of the organ from that by a central authority is the best possible one at present. It was always debatable if the priority should be given to a sick person who needs the organ with the possibility of a poorer outcome or it should be given to a relatively healthy person with a better prospect of good result. It is always a debatable point if an alcoholic with cirrhosis liver due to his habits should be a recipient of a liver transplant. Can a mentally challenged person come in the list for receiving organ? Can a person serving a prison sentence be the one for whom the organ is given. It is better that medical profession should not sit on moral judgment about preventable disease or moral issues.

11. Confidentiality of Donor and Recipient

It is prudent to maintain confidentiality about the donor and the recipients in a brain dead transplant program. But it is very often not possible as the public attention often identifies the donor and recipient from the news coverage of this selfless act of a grieving family. The donor family may like to know about the recipients in whose body their dear ones organs continue to live. This can lead to development of special bonding with positive results. On the negative side, it has been seen that the donor family contacts recipient families for financial support which is against the spirit of an altruistic action.

12. Brain Dead Minors and Mentally Challenge

The issue of minors and mentally challenged brain dead donors may not be a problem as live donation. This is because the issue of consenting will not arise as the consent is given by the legal heirs or guardians. But whether the allocation of the organ from a minor to another minor or an adult has to be thought off.

13. Donor Card Issues

The procedure of having donor cards identifies the presumed wish of a person when he was alive and helps in organ harvesting if he becomes brain dead. However, the consent of the immediate family members will be needed and the transplantation cannot be conducted if there is a wish against that by the near ones. In a big country like India follow-up of a person who has a donor card is a Herculean task to carry out the wish of the person. There is an argument if the person takes a donor card on an impulse and changes his decision later, the avenues for the opting out are not very clear in India.

14. Marginal or Suboptimal Organs

There is an ethical dilemma when the available organ is marginal or suboptimal. The recipient has to be fully aware of the use of this non-ideal organ and they should be provided with full information of the possible risks and benefits of using this. The incidence of delayed function and primary nonfunction is definitely greater with the use of a marginal donor. If the potential recipient rejects an offer of this non ideal organ where will they be in the allocation list?

Thus there are many ethical challenges in organising an active brain dead donation program in India. The wide disparity in education, financial status, and medical facilities available and public perception needs a constant educational process to improve the brain dead organ transplantation program in India. With the Governmental support in facilitating legal processes the program will spread across India, thus providing much needed organs for transplantation.

Further Reading

1. Adithyan GS, Mariappan M. Factors that determine deceased organ transplantation in India. Ind J Transplant. 11:26–30 (2017).

2. Ethics of organ donation in Biomedical Ethics. Olinda Timms. Reed Elsevier India Pvt Ltd, (2016).

3. George M. Aboun. Ethical Issues in Organ Transplantation. Med Princ Pract 12:54–69 (2003).

4. Lakshmi Kumar. Brain death and care of the organ donor. Journal of Anaesthesiology Clinical Pharmacology 32 (2016).

5. Palaniswamy V, Sadhasivam S, Selvakumaran C, et al. Organ donation after brain death in India: A trained intensivist is the key to success. Indian J Crit Care Med 20:593 (2016).

6. Robert Sells. Incentives for Organ Donation: Some Ethical Issues. Annals Of Transplantation, Vol. 9, No. 1, pp. 23–24 (2004).

7. Sanjay Nagral, J Amalorpavanathan. Deceased organ donation in India: where do we go from here? Ind. Journal of Medical Ethics Vol 11/3, 162–166 (2014).

8. Sanjay Nagral. Organ Transplantation: Ethical issues and the Indian scenario. Ind J Med Ethics. Vol 9/ 2, 41–43 (2001).

9. Shroff S, Rao S, Kurian G, Suresh S. Organ donation and transplantation—the Chennai experience in India. Transplant Proc 39:714–8 (2007).

10. Shroff S. Legal and ethical aspects of organ donation and transplantation. Ind J Urol 25:348–55 (2009).

11. Singh S, Kumar S, Dasgupta S et al. A single centre experience of kidney transplantation from donation after circulatory death: Challenges and scope in India. Ind. J Nephrol 27:205–209 (2017).

Principle, Ethics and Basic Skills of Counselling

Ameya Sunil Mahajan

INTRODUCTION

What is Counselling?

Counselling is an important skill which we need to understand and practice regularly while working as social worker. Need and method of counselling differs depending on the setting like hospitals, blood banks, school, de-addiction centre.

Counselling is a scientific process where a person who is having difficulties or problems (known as client) seeks professional help from person who is equipped with professional skills of counselling (known as counsellor)

Counselling is a continuous and time-bound process where a client seeks professional help to solve his/her problems. It is not easy process at all because there is need to maintain trust and purposeful and professional relationship between client and counsellor.

Now we will try to understand **Basic counselling skills** required for social workers.

Communication

Communication is an important skill required for counselling. In the initial phase when client approach to social worker to seek professional help need to maintain trust to the client and it will help to maintain professional and purposeful relationship.

Active Listening

Social worker who is playing role of counsellor has to be active listener. When client disclosed his/her problems with trust, it is necessary that being counsellor we have to listen actively and encourage client to discuss more on his/her issues, counsellor will be able to understand magnitude of the problems and its dimensions.

Empathy

Empathy is one of the most important skills that we need to practice consciously. Social worker needs to believe in empathy rather than sympathy. Empathy towards client helps us to see his/her problems in his/her perspective.

Clarification

While conducting session with client, a counsellor needs to be active listener, if required clarify what client has disclosed. Clarification will help counsellor to understand issue with clarity and accordingly will develop plans with the help of client. Timely clarification is very important to avoid confusion.

Effective Questioning Skills

Counsellor needs to understand that there should be effective questioning while conducting a session with client. It should be fine blending of open-ended and close-ended questions. Frame questions in such a way so that counsellor will get maximum information without taking much time.

Reflection

After every session counsellor needs to take down his/her notes need to maintain record in the form of case study and constantly need to reflect on it. This reflection process will help counsellor to get analytical picture of client problems/issues. It is necessary to reflect after every session with client and maintain records.

Observation

Observation is very important skill which a counsellor should inculcate. Observation of client's verbal and non-verbal communication will help to understand physical and mental status of the client. Sometimes during session on sensitive issues client suddenly becomes silent but we need to understand that silence also speaks many things. This observation needs to be documented to understand the behaviour of client during session and changes happen in the client as the session progresses gradually.

Ethics in Counselling

Ethics are set of rules or customs which are required for professional. Each profession having ethics needs to practice consciously. A counsellor needs to follow certain ethics while dealing with client.

Dignity

Each individual is having dignity and counsellor needs to maintain that dignity while dealing with client. Respect the rights of the client, also give his/her space in the process of counselling

Confidentiality

Important ethics needs to practice by counsellor to maintain confidentiality about his client and maintain trust among the client that whatever information disclosed by the client during counselling session will remain confidential and not get disclosed to anyone. Need to respect the right to confidentiality of the client.

Non-judgemental Attitude

Counsellor needs to maintain non-judgemental attitude while doing session with client. Counsellor should not be biased towards his client. Non-judgemental attitude will help counsellor to understand client in fair manner.

Informed Consent

Counselling is a process where counsellor and client are maintaining purposeful and professional relationship. It is necessary for the counsellor to take consent from the client for which he/she seeks professional help.

Counsellor needs to practice counselling in his/her setting actively and constant and conscious practice will help social worker to get command on it.

Law, Rules, Regulation and Guidelines

1. Salient Feature of THOA 1994 Amendments and Rules
2. Information on Zonal Transplant Coordination Centre, Mumbai
3. Formation and Functioning of ZTCC Pune
4. Police NOC in Organ Donation
5. SOP for Police No Objection Certification Case of Medicolegal Cases
6. Financial Assistance for Poor Patients
7. Maharashtra Government Resolutions

   Annexure

Salient Feature of THOA 1994 Amendments and Rules

Astrid Lobo Gajiwala and Sujata Ashtekar

The Transplantation of Human Organs Act, 1994

The Transplantation of Human Organs (Amendment) Act, 2011

The Transplantation of Human Organs and Tissues Rules, 2014

INTRODUCTION

The Transplantation of Human Organs Act (THOA), 1994 came into force on 4th February, 1995 in the States of Goa, Himachal Pradesh and Maharashtra and all the Union Territories.[1] Thereafter, it was adopted by all the States except the States of Jammu and Kashmir and Andhra Pradesh which have their own legislation.

This Act provided for "the regulation of removal, storage, and transplantation of human organs for therapeutic purposes and for the prevention of commercial dealings in human organs and for matters connected therewith or incidental thereto" (Long Title, THOA, 1994). It made the buying and selling of human organs a punishable offence.

The concept of brain stem death is recognised for the first time in this Act. It is defined as "the stage at which all functions of the brain stem have permanently and irreversibly ceased" [Chapter I, 2(d), THOA, 1994]. It also specified the requirements for certification of brain stem death. Thus it introduced a new definition of death. By declaring a person with brain stem death as dead it paved the way for the deceased donor organ donation programme in India.

In 2011, the Transplantation of Human Organs Act, 1994, was amended by The Transplantation of Human Organs (Amendment) Act, 2011, to include the regulation of tissues, and the amended Act was titled The Transplantation of Human Organs and Tissues Act (THOTA), 1994. In 2014, The Transplantation of Human Organs and Tissues (THOT) Rules, 2014, for the implementation of the amended Act were passed. The Government of Maharashtra adopted these Rules on 28 July, 2015.

The Ear Drums and Ear Bones (Authority for Use for Therapeutic Purposes) Act, 1989 and the Eyes (Authority for Use for Therapeutic Purposes) Act, 1982 are repealed under THOTA, 1994.

CONTENTS OF THE TRANSPLANTATION OF HUMAN ORGANS AND TISSUES ACT (THOTA), 1994

Chapter	Sections	Title
I	1–2	**Preliminary**
		1. Short title, application and commencement
		2. Definitions
II	3–9	**Authority for the Removal of Human Organs or Tissues or Both**
		3. Authority for the removal of human organs or tissues or both

4. Removal of human organs or tissues or both not to be authorized in certain cases

5. Authority for removal of human organs or tissues or both in case of unclaimed bodies in hospital or prison

6. Authority for removal of human organs or tissues or both from bodies sent for post-mortem examination for medicolegal or pathological purposes

7. Preservation of human organs or tissues or both

8. Savings

9. Restrictions on removal and transplantation of human organs or tissues or both

III	10–12	**Regulation of Hospitals**

10. Regulation of hospitals conducting the removal, storage or transplantation of human organs or tissues or both

11. Prohibition of removal or transplantation of human organs or tissues or both for any purpose other than therapeutic purposes

12. Explaining effects, etc. to donor and recipient

IV	13	**Appropriate Authority**

13-A. Advisory Committees to advise Appropriate Authority 13-B Powers of Appropriate Authority

V	14–17	**Registration of Hospitals**

14. Registration of hospitals engaged in removal, storage, and transplantation of human organs or tissues or both

14-A. Registration of Tissue bank

15. Certificate of registration

16. Suspension or cancellation of registration

17. Appeals

VI	18–22	**Offenses and Penalties**

18. Punishment for removal of human organ without authority

19. Punishment for commercial dealings in human organs

19-A. Punishment for illegal dealings in human tissues

20. Punishment for contravention of any other provisions of this Act

21. Offences by companies

22. Cognizance of offences

VII	23–25	**Miscellaneous**

23. Protection of action taken in good faith

24. Power to make rules

25. Repeal and savings

AUTHORISATION AND CONSENT FOR ORGAN AND TISSUE RETRIEVAL

Chapter I, section 2 of THOTA, 1994, provides definitions for the following; advertisement, Appropriate Authority, Authorisation Committee, brain stem death, deceased person, donor, hospital, human organ, human organ retrieval centre, minor, near relative, payment, recipient, registered medical practitioner, therapeutic purposes, tissue, Tissue Bank, transplantation and transplant co-ordinator.

Notable amendments in the definitions of the Principal Act are the introduction of 'Human Organ Retrieval Centre' in recognition of the organ and tissue donations that can occur in any hospital, including those that are not registered as transplant hospitals; "transplant co-ordinator" in recognition of the need for trained personnel to handle the many processes and procedures involved in organ and tissue donation from deceased donors; and "tissue" and Tissue Bank" to address a lacuna in the existing regulations and include tissues within the ambit of the Act. The amended definitions have also expanded the definition of "near relative" to include grandparents and grandchildren in addition to the previous spouse, children, parents and siblings.

Chapter II of THOTA, 1994, describes the conditions of consent and the authorities responsible for donation and removal of human organs and tissues for transplantation from living and deceased donors. It permits the donation of organs and tissues by the person lawfully in possession of the body of a deceased person "in whom permanent disappearance of all evidence of life occurs, by reason of brain stem death or in a cardiopulmonary sense, at any time after live birth has taken place" [Chapter I, 2(e)]. Thus it declares a brain stem dead person as deceased or dead and allows the donation of organs and tissues after both cardiac death and brain stem death.

This chapter permits any person above 18 years to pledge to donate their organs after death for therapeutic purposes, by expressing their wish in writing, in the presence of two or more witnesses at least one of whom is a near relative [Chapter II, 3(2), THOTA, 1994]. The format of the pledge is detailed in Form 7 of the THOT Rules, 2014. The person in lawful possession of the body can then give consent provided there is no reason to believe that the donor had subsequently revoked his/her pledge.

In the absence of a pledge, the person in lawful possession of the body can give consent for organ donation provided that there is no objection from any near relative of the deceased [Chapter II, 3(3), THOTA, 1994]. If the deceased brain stem dead person is a minor then either of the parents or any near relative authorised by the parent can give consent for organ donation [Chapter II, 3(7), THOTA, 1994 and 5(4) (d) THOT Rules, 2014].

Organs can be recovered only by a registered medical practitioner who is registered to do so. Tissues may be retrieved by registered medical practitioners with the exception of corneas which may be enucleated by qualified technicians [Chapter II, 3(4), THOTA, 1994].

Before retrieving the organs from a deceased donor it is the duty of the registered medical practitioner to confirm that life is extinct, or when brain stem death has occurred, that it has been certified as per the law [Chapter II, 3(5), THOTA, 1994].

Before undertaking the removal or transplantation of any human organ the registered medical practitioner must explain, in such manner as may be prescribed, all possible effects, complications and hazards connected with the removal and transplantation to the donor and the recipient respectively [Chapter III 12, THOTA, 1994].

BRAIN STEM DEATH CERTIFICATION

Brain stem death can only be certified by a Board of four medical experts consisting of the following:

i. The doctor in charge of the hospital in which brain stem death has occurred;

ii. An independent specialist doctor nominated by the registered medical practitioner specified in clause (i), from a panel of names approved by the Appropriate Authority and who is not connected with the transplant;

iii. A neurologist or a neurosurgeon to be nominated by the registered medical practitioner specified in clause (i), from the panel of names approved by the Appropriate Authority;

iv. The registered medical practitioner treating the person whose brain stem death has occurred.

If the neurologist or neurosurgeon is not available, the registered medical practitioner specified in clause (i) may nominate a registered medical practitioner, being a surgeon or a physician, and an anaesthetist or intensivist to certify brain stem death, subject to the condition that they are not members of the transplant team for the concerned recipient [Chapter II, 3(6), THOTA, 1994].

The process and criteria for brain stem death certification is given in Form 10 of the THOT Rules, 2014.

ORGAN AND TISSUE DONATION IN SPECIAL CIRCUMSTANCES

1. Unclaimed Bodies

In cases of unclaimed bodies in hospitals or prisons, if the body is not claimed within forty-eight hours from the time of death of the concerned person, then the person in charge of the hospital or prison or their authorised representative, can authorise organ donation. However, authorisation for donation cannot be given if there is reason to believe that any near relative of the deceased person is likely to claim the body, even if they have not come forward to claim the body within the specified time [Chapter II, 5(1) & (2), THOTA, 1994].

2. Medicolegal Cases

The body of a person is sent for post-mortem in medicolegal cases and for pathological purposes. A medicolegal case is declared when a person dies in an accident or any other unnatural cause. The donation of organs and tissues in these cases can only take place if they do not jeopardise the determination of the cause of death. Thus the competent authority must certify that the organs and tissues to be donated will not be required for the purpose for which the body has been sent for post-mortem, and give permission for their retrieval for therapeutic purposes (THOTA Chapter II, 6). When donations occur in medicolegal cases since a post-mortem is involved, efforts must be made to minimise inconvenience and delay in handing the body to the relatives for the funeral rites.

The procedure for the donation of organs or tissues in medicolegal cases is defined in THOT Rules 2014 (6).

1. After the authority for removal of organs or tissues, as also the consent to donate organs from a brain stem dead donor are obtained, the request is made by the registered medical practitioner of the hospital to the Station Superintendent of Police or Deputy Inspector General of the area either directly or through the police post located in the hospital to facilitate timely retrieval of organs or tissue from the donor. A copy of such a request should also be sent to the designated post-mortem doctor of the area simultaneously.

2. It shall be ensured that, by retrieving organs, the determination of the cause of death is not jeopardised.

3. The medical report in respect of the organs or tissues being retrieved shall be prepared at the time of retrieval by the retrieving doctor(s) and shall be taken on record in post-mortem notes by the registered medical practitioner doing post-mortem.

4. Wherever it is possible, attempt should be made to request the designated post-mortem doctor or registered medical practitioner, even beyond office timing, to be present at the time of organ or tissue retrieval.

5. In case a private retrieval hospital is not doing post-mortem, they shall arrange transportation of the body along with medical records, after organ or tissue retrieval, to the designated post-mortem centre and the post-mortem centre shall undertake the post-mortem of such cases on priority, even beyond office timing, so that the body is handed over to the relatives with least inconvenience.

3. Living Donors

The donation of organs is permitted from living donors under certain conditions. However, no organs or tissues can be removed from a minor before his/her "except in the manner as may be prescribed," or from a mentally challenged person [Chapter II, 9(1), THOTA, 1994].

Living donors are classified as related [a donor is a near relative] and unrelated donor [other than near relative] [Chapter II, 9(1), THOTA, 1994].

3.1. Related Living Donors

A near relative is defined as a spouse, parent, sibling, child, grandparents, grandchild of the recipient [Chapter I, 2(i), THOTA, 1994].

3.1.1. Swap transplantation

When a near relative living donor is medically incompatible with the recipient, the pair is permitted to do a swap transplant with another related unmatched donor and recipient pair where there is biological compatibility. Prior approval of the Authorisation Committee of the State is mandatory for a "swap transplantation". Such transplantations can only occur when the living donors are near relatives of the recipients [Chapter II, 9(3-A), THOTA, 1994].

3.1.2. Foreign nationals

Organ and tissue donation between a living donor and a foreign national can only take place if they are near relatives as defined by THOTA, 1994. Prior approval of the Authorisation Committee is mandatory [Chapter II, 9(1-A), THOTA, 1994].

When the proposed donor or the recipient is a foreign national:

a. A senior Embassy official of the country of origin has to certify the relationship between the donor and the recipient as per Form 21; in case a country does not have an Embassy in India, the certificate of relationship, in the same format, must be issued by the Government of that country;

b. The Authorisation Committee shall examine the cases of all Indian donors consenting to donate organs to a foreign national (who is a near relative), including a foreign national of Indian origin, with greater caution and such cases should be considered rarely on a case-to-case basis. (20, THOT Rules, 2014).

3.2. Unrelated Living Donors

Living donors who are not near relatives but are willing to donate organs to the recipients "by reason of affection or attachment towards the recipient or for any other special reasons," can do so only after obtaining the approval of the Authorisation Committee, established by the State under THOTA, 1994 [Chapter II, 9(3), THOTA, 1994]. In such circumstances the Authorisation Committee evaluates that there is no commercial transaction between the recipient and the donor. Factors such as the donor's relationship with the recipient, the authenticity of the link between the donor and the recipient, the reasons for the donation, the financial status of the donor and the recipient, and any strong views or disagreement or objection of near relatives of the donor may be considered [7(3), THOT Rules, 2014].

Living Woman Donors

In case the donor is a woman greater precautions must be taken to ensure that there is no coercion to donate. The donor's identity and independent consent should be confirmed in a confidential environment in the absence of the recipient and relatives.

REGISTRATION OF HOSPITALS AND TISSUE BANKS

The registration and regulation of hospitals and facilities conducting the removal, storage or transplantation of human organs or tissues or both, is described in Chapter III of THOTA, 1994. The registrations of transplant hospitals, NTORCs and tissue banks are valid for five years and must be renewed as required.

1. Transplant Hospitals

THOTA, 1994, provides for the registration of hospitals claiming to have the necessary competence and facilities to perform particular organ transplantations. This is a regulatory measure intended to protect the interests of patients. Hospitals intending to do transplants must register with the Appropriate Authority which is set up by the State Government/ Central Government in the case of Union Territories. Approvals are granted only after the institutions fulfil certain technical, infrastructural and medical requirements. The registration is renewed every five years.

Thus only hospitals registered under THOTA, 1994, can conduct or associate with, or help in, the removal, storage or transplantation of any human organ or tissue or both [Chapter III 10 (1)(a), THOTA, 1994]. However, the eyes and ears (ear drums and ear bones) may be removed by authorised persons (registered medical practitioner, or in the case of enucleation of cornea, a qualified technician) from the deceased donor at any place [Chapter III 10(2), THOTA, 1994]. The Rules, 2014 (26) describe the conditions and standards including experts and their qualifications, necessary for granting registration for organ and tissue transplantation centres. An application for registration of a hospital to carry out organ or tissue transplantation other than cornea must be submitted to the Appropriate Authority in Form 12 [24 (1), Rules, 2014].

Organs and tissues may be retrieved only for therapeutic purposes [Chapter III, 11, THOTA, 1994].

2. Non-Transplant Retrieval Centres (NTORCs)

The THOT Rules, 2014, make provision for organ and tissue donation from non-transplant hospitals [24 (1) (iii), Rules, 2014]. All hospitals with intensive care units (ICUs) and operation theatres have the potential to retrieve organs even if they may not have the facility to perform transplants. THOTA, 1994 permits such hospitals to be recognised as NTORCs by the Appropriate Authority. Applications must be made in Form 13 which specifies the infrastructure, personnel and equipment required to diagnose and maintain brain stem dead persons, and to retrieve and transport organs and tissues, including the facility for their temporary storage [27 (1) THOT Rules, 2014]. Organs retrieved from NTORCs are distributed to patients from transplant hospitals according to the State waiting lists.

All hospitals registered as transplant centres automatically qualify as retrieval centres.

3. Tissue Banks

The Rules, 2014,26 (2) and 28, describe the conditions and standards necessary for granting registration for tissue banks. The infrastructure, personnel and equipment required for the registration of tissue banks other than eye banks is specified in Form 14 (THOT Rules, 2014), and for eye banks and corneal retrieval and transplantation centres, are described in Form 15 (THOT Rules, 2014).

4. Transplant Co-ordinators

It is mandatory for all hospitals, whether registered for transplant or retrieval of organs, to appoint transplant co-ordinators whose qualification and role are defined in the THOT Rules, 2014, (29).

The "transplant co-ordinator" is defined as a person appointed by the hospital for co-ordinating all matters relating to removal or transplantation of human organs or tissues or

both and for assisting the authority for removal of human organs or tissues or both.

The transplant coordinator shall be an employee of the registered hospital and must have the following qualifications:
a. Graduate of any recognised system of medicine; or
b. Nurse; or
c. Bachelor's degree in any subject and preferably Master's degree in Social Work or Psychiatry or Sociology or Social Science or Public Health.

The transplant coordinator shall counsel and encourage the family members or near relatives of the deceased person to donate human organs and/or tissues including eye or cornea and coordinate the process of donation and transplantation.

It is the duty of the ICU registered medical practitioner to approach the relatives of the potential deceased donor in consultation with the transplant coordinator, to determine if the deceased individual had signed an organ and/or tissue donor pledge, or revoked the same. In the absence of a pledge the registered medical practitioner in consultation with the transplant coordinator must make the near relative or person in lawful possession of the body, aware of the option to authorise or decline the donation of such human organs or tissues or both which can be used for therapeutic purposes, including eye or cornea. Declaration or authorisation to this effect must be ascertained as per Form 8 [5(b), THOT Rules, 2014].

REGULATORY AND ADVISORY BODIES

The law defines regulatory and advisory bodies for monitoring transplantation activities.

1. Appropriate Authority

The Central (for Union Territories) or State government by notification appoints one or more of its officers as Appropriate Authorities for the purposes of this Act. The Appropriate Authority inspects and grants registration to hospitals for transplantation or retrieval of organs and tissues. She/he enforces required standards for hospitals and tissue banks and conducts regular inspections of these facilities. She/he examines the quality of transplantations and the follow-up of medical care to organ recipients and in the case of living donations, the living donor. She/he is required to investigate any complaints regarding breach of the provisions of the THOTA, 1994 and the THOT Rules, 2014, Act, and take appropriate action [Chapter IV, 13, THOTA, 1994]. For the purpose of this Act, she/he has all the powers of a civil court under the code of Civil Procedure 1908 to summon any person, request documents and issue search warrants when there is violation of this Act or the Rules made thereunder [Chapter IV, 13-B, THOTA, 1994].

2. Advisory Committee

The Advisory Committee is constituted by the Central and State Governments as the case may be, and consists of administrative, legal and medical experts in the field as well as social workers and a representative from non-government organisations, who shall aid and advise the Appropriate Authority to discharge its functions.

3. Authorization Committee

The Authorization Committee regulates the donation of organs from living donors by reviewing each case to ensure that the living donor is not exploited for monetary considerations and to prevent commercial dealings in transplantation. Proceedings of the Authorization Committees have to be video recorded and decisions notified within 24 hours of the application. Appeals against the decision of the Authorisation Committees may be made in writing to the State or Central Governments as applicable, within 30 days of receiving the order. A copy of the order appealed against must also be submitted [33, THOT Rules, 2014].

In Maharashtra the Director, Directorate of Health Services, is the Appropriate Authority and the Director, Directorate of Medical Education and Research is the Chairperson of the State Authorisation Committee which regulates hospitals doing less than twenty-five organ transplants in a year. Hospitals performing more than twenty-five organ transplants in a year are permitted to have their own Authorisation Committees [11 (3), THOT Rules, 2014].

NETWORKS

The THOT Rules, 2014, require the Central Government to establish National, Regional or State human organ and tissue removal and storage networks which are linked to each other and hospitals, organ and tissue matching laboratories and tissue banks in their area [31 (1) – (3), THOT Rules, 2014].. The apex network, the National Human Organ and Tissue Organisation (NOTTO) has been established at Delhi. Five Regional Organ and Tissue Transplant Organisations (ROTTO) have been established at Chandigarh, Chennai, Guwahati, Kolkata and Mumbai. State Organ and Tissue Transplant Organisations (SOTTO) are being set up in States that have adopted THOTA, 1994.

According to the Rules 2014, the networking organisations shall coordinate retrieval, storage, transportation, matching, allocation and transplantation of organs and tissues and shall develop norms and standard operating procedures for such activities and for tissues to the extent possible [31 (5)]. They shall also undertake Information, Education and Communication (IEC) activities for promotion of deceased organ and tissue donation [31 (11)] and maintain registries for organ and tissue donation and transplantation [31 (12)].

OFFENCES AND PENALTIES

Punishment for removal of organ without authority, making or receiving payment for supplying human organs or contravening any other provisions of the Act have been made very stringent in order to serve as a deterrent for such activities. Fines may extend to twenty-five lakh and prison terms up to 5 years depending on the offence.

The Act makes the offence of organ trading non-cognisable. In other words, the police cannot look into complaints of organ trading independently but must wait for a complaint to be made by the Appropriate Authority set up under the Act or by an officer authorised by it or by an individual who has given prior notice of not less than 60 days to the Appropriate Authority (Chapter VI, 22, THOTA, 1994).

MISCELLANEOUS

1. The cost for deceased donor management, retrieval of organs or tissues, their transportation and preservation shall not be borne by the donor family but may be borne by the recipient, institution, government, NGO or society as decided by the State Government or Union Territory Administration (9, Rules, 2014).

2. Hospitals are required to update their websites with regard to the total number of transplantations done along with reasonable detail for each transplantation. The data must be accessible to authorised persons in the respective State Governments and the Central Governments [32 (3), THOT Rules, 2014].

3. The identity of people in databases must not be put in the public domain and measures must be taken to ensure the security of all collected information [32 (11), THOT Rules, 2014].

FORMS SPECIFIED IN THE TRANSPLANTATION OF HUMAN ORGANS AND TISSUES RULES, 2014

Form 1: For Organ or Tissue Donation from Identified Living Near related Donor (To be completed by him/her)

Form 2: For Organ or Tissue Donation by Living Spousal Donor (To be completed by him/her)

Form 3: For Organ or Tissue Donation by Other than Near Relative Living Donor (To be completed by him/her)

Form 4: For Certification of medical Fitness of Living Donor (To be given to the Registered Medical Practitioner)

Form 5: For Certification of Genetic relationship of Living Donor with Recipient (To be filled by the Head of the Pathology Laboratory certifying relationship)

Form 6: For Spousal Living Donor (To be filled by the competent authority and Authorisation Committee of the hospital/District/State in case of foreigners)

Form 7: For Organ or Tissue Pledging (To be filled by an individual of age 18 years or above)

Form 8: For Declaration cum Consent (To be filled by the near relative or lawful possessor of the brain stem dead person)

Form 9: For Unclaimed Body in a Hospital or Prison (To be completed by person in lawful possession of the unclaimed body)

Form 10: For Certification of Brain stem Death (To be filled by the Board of medical experts certifying brain stem death)

Form 11: Application for Approval of Transplantation from Living Donor (To be completed by the proposed recipient and the proposed living donor)

Form 12: Application for Registration of Hospital to carry out Organ or Tissue Transplantation other than Cornea (To be filled by the head of the institution)

Form 13: Application for Registration of Hospital to carry out Organ or Tissue Retrieval other than Eye/Cornea Retrieval (To be filled by the head of the institution)

Form 14: Application for Registration of Tissue Banks other than Eye Banks (To be filled by the head of the institution)

Form 15: Application for Registration of Eye Bank, Corneal Transplantation Centre, Eye Retrieval Centre under Transplantation of Human Organs Act

Form 16: Certificate of Registration for Performing Organ/Tissue Transplantation/Retrieval and/or Tissue Banking

Form 17: Certificate of Renewal of Registration (To be given by the Appropriate Authority on the Letterhead)

Form 18: Certificate by the Authorisation Committee of Hospital/District / State where the Transplantation has to take place. (To be issued on the letterhead)

Form 19: Certificate by Competent Authority (For Indian near relative, other than spouse, cases)

Form 20: Verification Certificate in respect of Domicile Status of Recipient or donor (To be issued by Tehsildar or any other authorised officer for the other than near relative donor or recipient, if they do not belong to the State where the transplant hospital is located)

Form 21: Certificate of relationship Between Donor and Recipient in Case of Foreigners (To be issued by Embassy concerned).

Information on Zonal Transplant Coordination Centre, Mumbai

SK Mathur

Zonal Transplant Coordinator Centre, Mumbai is a not-for-profit, government formed coordinating agency. It is formed in December 2000 to coordinate, monitor and promote deceased organ donation in Mumbai and suburb. It is registered with charity commissioner's office.

Human Organ Transplantation Act was passed in 1994 in India and it was adopted by Maharashtra in 1995. In the meeting which was called by Directorate of Health Services to discuss about implementation of deceased donor programme in Maharashtra on 24th May 1995 it was proposed by the experts present (Late Dr V N Acharya, Dr A Kriplani, Dr GB Daver and Dr SK Mathur) that the regulation of transplant should be done at three levels.

1. There should be central coordinating body at state level incorporating Appropriate Authority and authorisation committee and others.

2. There can be a Coordinating body formed by an NGOs such as National Kidney Foundation and other like-minded bodies.

3. Registered Transplant Hospitals where organ transplants and Organ Retrievals will be done.

In Maharashtra, Directorate of Health Services is Appropriate Authority and Directorate of Medical Education and Research is Authorisation. The Appropriate Authority gave registrations to the hospitals for retrieval and transplants of the organs.

On 9th July, 1999, Maharashtra Government issued Government Resolution (GR) for the implementation of deceased donor transplant programme in state of Maharashtra.

This GR of 1999 also notified the formation of the, "Maharashtra Confederation for Organ Transplant" (MCFOT) was formed as state level advisory body with the aims to promote deceased donor transplant programme in the state, to cooperate with the Appropriate Authority for implementation of deceased donor programme and to coordinate with the city level coordinating agencies, [ZTCCs] and to create awareness about organ donation.

The 1st meeting of MCFOT was held on 31st August 1999 under the Chairmanship of Mr TC Benjamin, Secretary, Medical Education and Drug Department with Fig. 2.1 agenda.

The Zonal Transplant Coordination Centres were proposed at four cities, Mumbai, Pune, Nagpur and Aurangabad. Presently all the four ZTCCs are functioning efficiently (Fig. 2.1).

Mumbai Zonal Transplant Coordination Centre, was the first ZTCC which was created by MCFOT in its meeting held on 31st March, 2000 and started functioning in the same year under the chairmanship of Mr, Julio Reberio IPS (Retd.) and Dr Vatsala Trivedi, HOD (Urology), LTM Medical College and Hospital was nominated as Secretary. First meeting was held on 18th Dec. 2000 under the

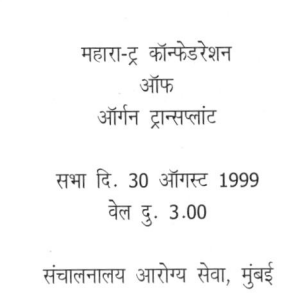

महारा-ट्र कॉन्फेडरेशन
ऑफ
ऑर्गन ट्रान्सप्लांट

सभा दि. 30 ऑगस्ट 1999
वेळ दु. 3.00

संचालनालय आरोग्य सेवा, मुंबई

AGENDA

1. To define the objective and the role of MAHARASHTRA CONFEDERATION FOR ORGANS TRANSPLANT.

2. To decide upon the exact role of ZTCCs at City level and progress made by ZTCC in the City of Mumbai.

3. To assess and progress made in the Cadaveric Transplant Programme by the recognised hospitals.

4. To consider recognition of certain hospitals for retrieval of organs only, as per the request received.

5. Any other point with the permission of the Chair.

Fig. 2.1: MCFOT 1st meeting

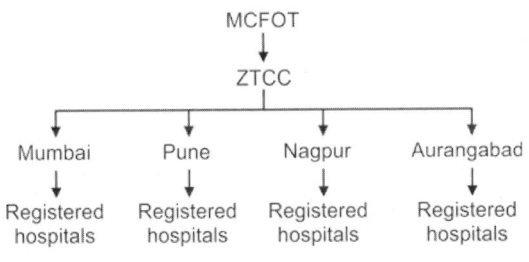

Fig. 2.2

Chairmanship of Mr. Julio Reberio, 13 registered hospitals participated. Mrs Sujata Ashthekar became the first Hon. Transplant Coordinator with ZTCC Mumbai. In the year 2001, Memorandum of Association and Rules Regulations were framed and registered with Charity Commissioner. The Constitution of ZTCC Mumbai was subsequently amended in years 2005 and 2013.

Other ZTCCs followed similar memorandum, rules and regulations.

Composition of ZTCC, Mumbai

Members: All the registered Transplant Hospitals in Mumbai suburbs and Thane city are the members of the ZTCC, Mumbai. It is made mandatory for them by the State. Members of NGOs promoting organ donation are included.

A. Executive council: It consists of the following members:
- President [elected]
- Two Vice President [elected]
- Gen. Secretary [elected]
- Joint Secretary [elected]
- Treasurer

Chairpersons of expert subcommittees are also the members of executive council.

Meeting of executive council is held once a month.

B. Governing council: It consists of the following members:
- CEOs/Deans/Commandants of all recognized member hospitals.
- Representative from NGOs.
- Chairpersons of all expert committees
- Representative of State Appropriate Authority
- Invitee members.
- Meeting of Governing Council is held every three months.

C. General body: All members of various committees are the members of General Body.

The meeting of the general body is held once a year.

ZTCC formed expert committees for providing technical guidance. Experts members [one physician and one surgeon] of this committees are from all recognized institution and form subcommittee for each organ, e.g.
- Kidney and pancreas
- Liver
- Heart
- Bone marrow
- Cornea
- Skin and tissue bank
- Any other organ

There is a subcommittee of social workers and transplant coordinators.

The meeting of the expert committee is called by a chairperson as and when required.

Miscellaneous Subcommittee formed by the nomination.
- Internal audit committee
- Ethics committee

The Chairman and the Secretary are elected by individual committees.

The term of each committee is for three years.

The members have right to get re-nominated for totally 2 terms only.

ZTCC is an organization on par with international standards with the following main aims.
- To promote deceased donor [cadaver] transplant.
- Optimal use of all cadaveric available organs.
- To reach out to every needy waiting recipient with fair distribution of organs as per government guidelines.

Functions of ZTCC, Mumbai

- To maintain the common waiting list of needy recipients for each organ at the city level.
- To distribute the organ to the most suitable recipient as per the priority criteria given in the state guidelines.
- Co-ordinate all activities for procurement of organs.
- Organize awareness program for professionals as well as public to promote cadaver transplants.

Transplant registry: The ZTCC, Mumbai maintains the computerized waiting list blood group wise for each organ like kidney, liver, heart and lung as per the priority criteria given in the Maharashtra State guidelines. All the registered transplant hospitals send the information of the patients required cadaver organ in the prescribed form for listing. For kidney, each patient is given priority score as per the guidelines. Criteria for the score are like age of the patient, period on dialysis, waiting period with ZTCC, earlier graft failure, fistula failure, etc. For liver, priority is mainly as per the blood group and date of registration if there is no patient in super urgent category.

The patient's name is registered through hospital and the patients cannot get registered directly to the ZTCC. When the organ is available, the organ is offered to the patient only in the hospital from where it is registered with the ZTCC.

As on January 2018, there are 35 hospitals registered with ZTCC, Mumbai. There are approximately 3400 patients waiting for kidney, 280 for liver and 35 for heart and 5 patients for lungs.

Organ Distribution

When there is a brain death in the registered hospital in Mumbai and nearby suburb, the ZTCC, Mumbai is informed. The first kidney goes to the donor hospital patient having highest priority score in that blood group. The second kidney is offered to the patients on city waiting list as per the priority score. The liver is first offered to the patient listed in the super urgent category [this listing is done after the expert committee approval], if there is no super urgent category patient, then the liver is offered to the donor hospital. If there is no patient from the same blood group on the hospital list, then the liver is offered to the city waiting list.

The ZTCC co-ordinators contact hospital co-ordinators who inform the patients about the availability of the organ. The distribution report and reason for refusal are written and filed in the ZTCC office.

If there is no recipient in the city for any organ, then the organ is further offered to other ZTTCs in the state and then to Regional or National level through ROTTO-SOTTO [Regional and State Organ and Tissue Transplant Organisation].

Awareness and Promotional Activities

The ZTCC, Mumbai has been promoting organ donation by conducting various awareness activities.
- Pamphlet and Donor Card distribution—donor card pamphlet has mobile nos. which are contactable day and night.
- Putting up stall at community meetings. Ganesh Pandals, Navratri Utsav, Colleges, corporate, etc.

- Awareness talks—ZTCC representatives go to various places to give talks or power point presentation on organ donation. Like:
  - Various Social groups, e.g, Rotary club, Lions club, Mahila Mandals, Ganesh Pandals
  - Community gathering
  - Corporate offices
  - Religious places like temples, churches, Gurudwara
- Participate in Rallies, Marathon to promote organ donation
- Co-ordinate for role plays, street plays on organ donation with the help of college students, office workers.
- Newspaper reports, magazines—the ZTCC members have written articles in magazines to promote organ donation.
- Donor family felicitation is organised every year to appreciate and felicitate the family members of the brain dead donors for their noble contribution.

Training Programmes

We conduct CMES in the hospitals and for NTORCS to sensitize the professionals. Conduct training programme for MSWs/para-professionals.

Dr S K Mathur MS, FACS

HPB & Liver Transplantation Surgeon.

- Vice President & Ag Gen Sec ZTCC Mumbai
- Founder Member of MCFOT and ZTCC
- Member Govt of MH Committee for Liver Transplantation Guidelines

Former

- Professor of General & GI Surgery, Seth GS Medical College & KEM Hospital, Mumbai
- Professor and HOD, Gen & GI Surgery, TN Medical College and BYL Nair Hospital, Mumbai

Formation and Functioning of ZTCC Pune

Abhay Huprikar

The Govt of Maharashtra has established ZTCC to create awareness about organ donation among the people, and also to ensure fair distribution of organs in the concerned city. This committee maintains a list of patients who need organ transplant (who cannot get it from their relatives), and also collects the data about brain dead patients in the region. The ZTCC makes sure that all the patients get organs according to the waiting list. The ZTCC has offices in Pune, Mumbai, Aurangabad and Nagpur. All the hospitals which perform organ transplantation, work under the guidelines of this ZTCCs. As the Govt. wanted these bodies to be registered as trusts, the ZTCC Pune has been registered as a society under the Societies Registration Act, 1860 and as a public charitable trust under the Bombay Public Trusts Act, 1950 with the Charity Commissioner, Pune. The trust is also registered under the Income Tax Act, 1961. The ZTCC functions along strict parameters laid down by the MCFOT, State Dept. of Health in all respects and is subject to regular monitoring and monthly reporting to DHS and DMER.

The Pune ZTCC is run by a Managing Committee comprising of a Chairman, Vice Chairman, Secretary, Treasurer, other elected members, Ex-officio trustees representing Government Hospitals and invites from registered hospitals. The day-to-day working of the committee is undertaken by an executive central coordinator. Apart from the core

functions mentioned above, the ZTCC is actively involved in spreading awareness among the public as well as medical and paramedical personnel. This is a vital activity, as general awareness about organ donation is very poor in our society.

Once brain death is recognized, there are lots of processes to be carried out, if the donor or brain dead person has medicolegal case (case of injury or ailment); it also involves registering FIR with the police and post-mortem documentation. This requires time and joint efforts of police department, relatives of deceased person, and doctors. After completing all these procedures and transplantation surgeries, it will help bring back that smile on the face of two patients suffering from blindness, two patients with kidney failure on dialysis and one patient whose liver is not working, patients suffering from myocardiopathy does heart transplant. All these 6 patients will give blessings to the person—the donor because of whom they got that smile on their face.

Broad Functions of ZTCC Pune

- Every month we conduct managing committee meeting to discuss various issues and policies and take decisions accordingly
- Every year AGM will be conducted in month of September. (before 30th)
- After every 3 months all transplant coordinators meet to discuss issues about

deceased donor transplant and for good coordination among themselves

- We also have subcommittee working in different areas.
  A. Public awareness committee
  B. Liver subcommittee
  C. Website development committee
  D. Kidney, Pancreas and Multiviseral sub-committee

  For listing our patients for all organs, i.e. Heart, liver, kidney, pancreas, and multiviseral, we have cloud base system which has accurate listing, allocation and distribution. A mobile app. is given to all coordinators.

  From year 2013 our programme picked up in all over the region in all aspects; like we have increased no. of donations; awareness programme, filling up with donor cards, etc. We also have organized Training programme for Transplant Coordinators and CME for doctors at various places in Pune and other cities.

To improve organ donation rates in the city, the ZTCC Pune would like to put the following appeals to health care providers and society at large

i. Treating physicians and an intensivists and doctors should identify all brain stem deaths, and report to DHS and ZTCC.

ii. Expansion of accredited Brain Death Com-mittees to cover all relevant hospitals including NTORCS.

iii. In medicolegal (MLC) cases, the Police Department needs to be made more aware of the concept of brain death and the law so that valuable time is not lost in pro-cedures such as NOCs for organ retrieval.

iv. In MLC cases, the authorities should be requested to expedite autopsies to reduce the emotional hardship of the relatives.

v. All transplant professionals and involved coordinators/social workers should join in the efforts to increase social awareness.

vi. The public should be encouraged to sign and carry donor cards.

Some Historical Aspect of ZTCC Pune

1997—First Kidney transplant—Pune Ruby Hall

2013—First liver transplant—Pune Ruby Hall

2016—First Kidney Pancreas transplant—DMH Hospital, Pune

2017—First heart transplant—Ruby Hall Clinic, Pune

Film On Organ Donation—"*Phirzindagi*"

Statistics of ZTCC Pune					
Year	No. of cadaver donor	Kidney trans-plant	Liver trans-plant	Com bined trans-plant	Heart trans-plant
2013	10	15	4		
2014	8	13	8		
2015	16	30	11		
2016	59	88 Kidney +Pancreas –1	58		
2017 (June)	29	42	28	1 KP	6

2 shared to ZTCC Mumbai

Achievements of ZTCC Pune

Not only the total number of brain dead patients. have increased but their conversion to number of transplants have increased (>60%).

Extremely good support from press, T.V., print media, general public.

Increase in Voluntary Donation.

Maharashtra got best state and Ruby Hall as best hospital. Award & Surekha Joshi as *Best Tx coordinator* at National Organ Donor Day at New Delhi given by Health minister at the programme by NOTTO.

Organ donation started very actively in Nasik, Solapur, Kolhapur under Pune ZTCC region

Government hospital did 4 donations and 1 kidney transplant with great motivation of Dean BJMC, Pune.

Police NOC in Organ Donation

Prakash Saindane

Organ donation is being increased day by day. Nevertheless there is huge gap between organ requirements and availability of organs. We need to eliminate the barriers of organ donation to increase numbers of donation and to meet the need of organs.

Brain stem death (BSD) occurs due to road traffic accidents (RTA), intracranial bleeding, haemorrhage, etc. Most of these cases are medicolegal cases (MLC). According to our protocols we need to take police NOC for removing organs in MLC. It is not required for non-MLC. Police NOC is given if the organs are not needed for post-mortem. It may be considered as a security for hospitals that are performing cadaver organ donation. Police takes Jabab (interview) of family members after hospital requisition for NOC. They do thoroughly inquest and after satisfaction of all necessary inquiries they issue an NOC.

As per the Transplantation of Human Organ Act 1994 (THOA) police NOC is not required but states have made their own protocols in implementation of the transplant program. Police NOC is one of the parts of these protocols.

The ideal guidelines say that donor hospital is supposed to inform to neighbourhood police station after declaration of brain dead after second set of apnoea is done. Police station is already having MLC record as the MLC is registered at admission by hospital. Neighbourhood/local police station is supposed to give police NOC. If the NOC is

getting this way, it would be very smooth and easier for hospital coordination team and it can save time, organ retrieval would not get delayed. The police who have to inquire and issue the NOC are always in dilemma that whether or not they have to issue the NOC, why NOC is needed from police. They suspect that issuing NOC may create problem for them if some legal complications arise over the time of period.

In my experience I have observed that police officials are not aware about organ donation and its process. They do not object organ donation but they are reluctant to issue NOC. They want organ donation but they do not want themselves to be grabbed in this process. It is because of lack of awareness of legalities, importance of organ donation and role of police in this regards.

Most of the brain dead cases are MLCs. Treating hospital registers MLC if it is road traffic accident (RTA) or sudden attack or unclear cause of death. The brain death occurs at treating hospital but accident may happen somewhere else. The first MLC is registered where the accident takes place; patient may be admitted at local hospital following by shifting another hospital for further advance treatment. Brain death occurs at second hospital. It does mean the concern police station where brain death is occurred differs from the police station where first MLC is registered. Neighbourhood police station says the first police station should issue NOC and first police station throws the ball in second police station's court.

There are no clear cut guidelines in issuing police NOC in organ donation. Police argue that where the requirement of such NOC is written in law or state guidelines and really nowhere clearly it is written. Transplant coordinator is answerless in this situation. Mumbai police commissioner had issued a circular in 2012 to procure the NOC as soon as hospital has approached the local police station but it is not very useful. In-charge police officers get transferred after a certain period and next officers are not aware about this circular. Transplant coordinator explains the same process in every case to everyone, after a long arguments and debate hospital gets NOC. This is a recurrent problem which Mumbai has been facing for a very long period.

Donor hospital and local coordinating team respects the donor family and try to make everything easier in all the processes. Family should not get trouble in their grief. We request police personnel to come to hospital for inquest and reporting. They can come and do documentation in hospital but mostly they prefer to call family to police station. Hospital team wish to have all the processes in hospital itself for avoiding family trouble but where getting NOC is a heavy exercise, does not want to make more barriers in process.

It is observed that there is no conceptual clarity about organ donation among police officials. They have significant concerns regarding completion of legal paperwork and formalities before being able to issue the NOC. That is why government should make a legal outline through government rules where they would feel secured and they would have written legal protocols to carry out the processing.

These are some hurdles in organ donation program. Awareness among all concerned people needs to be done; we need to have some firm government decisions, allocation of accountability of all individuals and departments need to be clarified. We need to look at organ donation as a social and noble cause.

SOP for Police No Objection Certification Case of Medicolegal Cases

Anirudh K Kulkarni

A police No Objection Certificate (NOC)/ intimation is required before retrieving organs only, if it is a medicolegal case.

Procedure for the transplant coordinator

1. After 1st set of tests (including the apnoea test) for brain stem death, and oral consent of the family for organ donation, intimate the concerned police station about the possibility of organ donation in the hospital.
2. After the 2nd set of tests for brain stem death is performed and brain death has been certified on Form No. 10 of the Transplantation of Human Organs and Tissue (THOT) Rules, 2014, and written consent for organ donation has been obtained, approach the nearest police station for a police NOC.
4. Give a letter from the donor hospital to the concerned police station requesting the police to conduct an inquest and give an NOC for organ donation. Forms No. 10 and 8 of the THOT Rules, 2014, must be attached with this letter and given to the police for their record.
5. Request the police to come to the hospital for recording the statement of the family members of the brain stem dead donor and their decision to donate organs and/or tissues.
6. The police will give an NOC for organ and/or tissue donation.
7. After obtaining the police NOC the donor will be shifted to operation theatre.

8. After the retrieval of solid organs, the body is shifted to the ICU for eye and skin retrieval if there is consent for the same.
9. Update the police about the retrieval, so that they can conduct further procedures like an inquest/punchnama.
10. After organ and/or tissue retrieval the body of the donor is handed over to the police for the post-mortem [PM] along with the clinical notes of the retrieval surgeon.
11. Accompany the family when the body is taken for the PM.
12. The PM authority verifies the consent of the family and Form No. 8, THOT Rules, 2014.
13. The PM authority also verifies other documents like the brain stem death certificate, police NOC, retrieval team's operative notes, etc.
14. After the PM is done, the authority will issue a death certificate which mentions organ and/or tissue donation.

Note

The organs and tissues retrieved after obtaining the consent of the family has to be clearly specified on the following:

1. Police statement
2. Police NOC
3. Report of the inquest *punchnama*
4. Operative notes of the retrieval surgeon.

Financial Assistance for Poor Patients

Ruchita Masurkar

Patients suffering from chronic diseases have major cost requirement towards the treatment. Such a big amount is difficult to raise even for a middle class family. Patient's life turns upside down not only physically but also mentally. This drains him/her off financially at the end of the treatment as the treatment is prolonged one. Patient's family has to shell out money through self and help of relatives and friends. It's really a difficult phase where not only the patient but the whole family is disturbed and when it comes to monetary arrangement for treatment it is a task for family to arrange funds.

Hospitals also help contribute towards treating patients in subsidized class. However, the flow of patients is so high that it is beyond the scope to extend the facility to larger number of patients. Hence the only hope for such families is to receive donations from trusts giving financial medical help. To receive these donations, many hospitals have social work department through which, these families are guided for fund raising and reference letters are offered.

For example, in Mumbai, major support of financial help towards medical treatment comes from trust giving financial medical aids. TATA Trusts, CM Fund, PM Fund, Being human foundation and temples trusts like Siddhivinayak, Shree Mahalaxmi, Haji Ali Darga, etc. They are the ones who support kidney transplant patients. All trusts have their own rules and regulations. Documents like ID proof, Ration card, Income Proof, NOC from hospital (Authorisation committee), Doctor's cost estimate on hospital letterhead along with Doctor's stamp, Electricity Bill and Bank Passbook are generally required while seeking financial aid.

Following are details of few trusts who help in Chronic Kidney Disease (CKD)

1. **Tata trusts:** The office is in Fort area, Mumbai and the trusts has major links with hospitals where patients can get guidance and references of the same. For more details one can go through TATA Trusts website http://www.tatatrusts.org/. Patient's kin has to submit above mentioned documents and personally visit trust office on weekdays.

2. **CM fund:** The application needs to be done directly at Mantralaya along with Doctor's cost estimate, Aadhar Card, Ration Card, Income Certificate, NOC from hospital (Authorisation committee).

3. **PM fund:** Patient's kin needs to contact MP Office and courier the details along with Member of Parliament Letter to PM Office, Delhi.

4. **Dr SHM Modi trusts:** The office is in Nariman Point, Mumbai. The application needs to be done along with above mentioned documents.

5. Temples trusts: Shree Mahalaxmi, Siddhi-vinayak, Babulnath, Haji Ali dargah.

Apart from above mentioned trusts, there are many other trusts (please check annexure enclosed) who support in small amounts to patients. Even though the amount is less, it proves to be valuable contribution for patients as the treatment is prolonged one. Post-kidney or any solid organ transplant, the patient would be on expensive medication for long time. Patients can apply to Jeevan Jyot Drug Bank in Tardeo, Mumbai for medicine at subsidised rates. These contribution from trusts helps motivate coordinators to form Social Work Department to help and guide families in need of financial help for their near and dear ones.

"Let's work together and contribute to save precious lives"...

Maharashtra Government Resolutions

Responsibilities of Hospitals Registered Under
Human Organ Transplant Act, 1994

GOVERNMENT OF MAHARASHTRA
PUBLIC HEALTH DEPARTMENT
Government Resolution No-Map 2012/C. R289/AROGYA-6
Mantralaya Mumbai 400032
Date: 13th Septmber 2012

Read: The Transplantation of Human Organs Act, 1994 and the Transplantation of Human Organs Rules 1995

Government Resolution

The Government is committed to streamlining the procedures for Organ Transplant in Maharashatra State. Being aware that a large number of patients are awaiting organ transplant and are dependent on authorized transplant centers, several orders have been issued including formation of the appropriate authority, functioning of authorization committee and so on.

1. It is now felt that in the current scenario where more hospitals are being registered as transplant centers, it becomes necessary to ensure that transparency, accountability, patient well-being and quality care are adequately taken care of. Also considering the fact that cadaver donation is done with altruistic motives and in a generous charitable manner as a willing contribution to society, it is necessary that cadaver donation be governed by transparency on all fronts to ensure that the sentiments of the donor's relatives are adequately respected. Hence, it is considered necessary that certain degree of accountability is also insisted upon. Considering this, the following orders regarding further responsibilities of registered transplant centers are issued.

2. All transplant centers shall maintain all transplant surgery records as required in the Act and Government Resolutions for a minimum period of ten years.

3. All transplant centers shall ensure the availability of a counselling department/wing to whom the task of counselling individuals involved in organ transplant is entrusted. This counselling department/wing should be staffed with personnel who are adequately trained. The assistance of NGOs professionally involved in counselling may be secured. In

the case of non-near relative live donors, the counselling department may assist in ensuring that there is no element of coercion or other pressure exerted on the donor and also assist in provision of post-operative counselling.

4. Each transplant centre shall designate a transplant coordinator in the hospital, who may be in-house on account of interest/expertise and their role may be defined by the hospital concerned. Transplant coordinator shall play the coordinating role in all matters relating to organ transplant on behalf of the hospital that they represent.

5. A transplant centre hospital shall not reveal the identity of the recipient or attract any form of media publicity earlier than the date of discharge of recipients. Even after discharge, while the positive aspects of organ donation may be highlighted to promote the cause of organ donation, neither should that details of the recipients nor should the ethics of the medical profession towards attracting publicity be compromised or violated in any manner.

6. In order to ensure transparency and accountability for the reason mentioned above, all transplant centre hospitals that wish to benefit from the cadaver transplant program are required to display the approximate range of cost of a transplant surgery by specifying the organ type on the website of the hospital and the website designated for this purpose by the Public Health Department.

By order and in the name of Governor.

13.9.2012

(T.C. Benjamin)
Additional Chief Secretary

Human Organ Transplant Act 1994
Declaration of brain death

GOVERNMENT OF MAHARASHTRA
PUBLIC HEALTH DEPARTMENT
Government Resolution No-Maapra-2012/C. R289/Health-6
Mantralaya Mumbai 400032
Date: 13th Septmber 2012

Read: The Transplantation of Human Organs Act, 1994 and the Transplantation of Human Organs Rules 1995

Government Resolution

It has been brought to the notice of the Government that Brain death is not declared promptly. Further, doubts have arisen in medical circles on the authority by which doctors may declare "Brain Death" whenever required. Several patients who are brain dead have been kept on life support system in the Hospitals needlessly, thereby delaying/pre-empting Organ Transplant to needy patients. It is also a fact that failure to declare brain death even when all the conditions for such a condition are evident, has led to prolonged but avoidable anxiety for the concerned family members and friends of the patients.

Due to lack of clarity on this issue and the optional nature of the current situation, it has become necessary to issue orders making it mandatory to declare "Brain Death" and certify it accordingly.

The following orders are therefore issued in the matter:

It is now made mandatory that whenever the medical condition (clinical and medical criteria prescribed) of a patient has reached a brain death stage, brain death certification shall be done by the authorized medical personnel and immediately thereafter the details of the brain death certification shall be conveyed to the Zonal Transplantation Co-ordination committee for distribution of the Organs.

The above order shall come into force in Hospitals which are registered under Human Organ Transplant Act 1994 and Non-transplant Organ Retrieval Centres in the state with immediate effect.

The procedures to be followed for declaring brain death and the authorized personnel for undertaking the same will be issued separately.

By order and in the name of the Governor

13.9.2012

(T.C. Benjamin)
Additional Chief Secretary

Procedure for the Declaration
of Brain Death

GOVERNMENT OF MAHARASHTRA
PUBLIC HEALTH DEPARTMENT
Government Resolution No-Maapra-2012/CR. 289/Health-6
Mantralaya Mumbai 400032
Date: 13th Septmber 2012

Read: The Transplantation of Human Organs Act, 1994 and the Transplantation of Human Organs Rules 1995

Government Resolution

1. Declaration for Brain Death has been made mandatory in Transplant Hospitals and in Non-transplant Organ retrieval centres registered under Human Organ Transplant Act 1994 by Appropriate Authority.

2. Whereas the Transplantation of Human Organs Act of 1994 (THO Act) and the Transplantation of Human Organs Rules, 1995 (THO Rules) are the only pieces of legislation available wherein brain death certification procedures have been elaborately laid down, it is hereby decided that the procedures outlined therein will also be adopted as brain death certification procedure in Maharashatra. This order will also elaborate on the above format to ensure its applicability to the state.

3. Form 8 of THO Act and Rules prescribed as the brain death certification format is to be utilised for any given situation requiring certification that a person is dead on account of permanent and irreversible cessation of all functions of the brain stem. The tests prescribed therein and findings required shall remain the same.

4. According to Form 8 of the said Act and Rules, when such certification is required, there shall be two medical examinations conducted by a team of Doctors after a minimum interval of six hours and the findings made based on the tests prescribed therein.

5. According to form 8 of the above Act and Rules, four Doctors are authorised to certify Brain death and this provision is clarified further, as under:

    i. Doctor No. 1 is the 'RMP in charge of the hospital in which brainstem death has occurred'.

    ii. Doctor No. 2 is the 'RMP (Physicians, Surgeons or Intensivists) nominated from the panel of names approved by the appropriate authority. Accordingly, a' panel of names shall be sent by Dean/Medical Superintendent/Medical Director to the Appropriate Authority, namely the Director of Health Services and on approval shall then be utilised as the panel from which a RMP shall be nominated for each brain death certification. Each hospital may determine its own procedure for this nomination.

    iii. Doctor No. 3 is 'Neurologist/Neuro-surgeon nominated from the panel of names approved by the Appropriate Authority'. Again, a panel of names shall be sent by the Dean/Medical Superintendent/Medical Director to the Appropriate Authority, namely the Director of Health Services and on approval shall then be utilised as the panel from which one specialist as in the category therein shall be nominated for each brain death certification. Each hospital may determine its own procedure for this nomination.

iv. Doctor No. 4 is the RMP treating the aforesaid person. This does not require any clarification and shall be the RMP/Doctor on duty treating the patient (No clearances are required from the Appropriate Authority in this category).

Note I: In the event of lack of authorised personnel in Category.

v. Above, in the NTORC hospital concerned, a request may be made to any other member of the panel from the Brain stem death committee of hospital registered under Human Organ Transplant Act by the Appropriate Authority.

vi. The 1st and 2nd Medical examination as defined in Form 8 of the THO rules shall be conducted by category (ii) and (iii) doctors from the panel approved by the appropriate authority.

By order and in the name of Governor

13.9.2012

(T.C. Benjamin)
Additional Chief Secretary

Criteria for Non-Transplant Centres to
Retrieve Organs from Brain Dead Persons

GOVERNMENT OF MAHARASHTRA
PUBLIC HEALTH DEPARTMENT
Government Resolution No-MAP-2012/CR. 289/Arogya-6
Mantralaya Mumbai 400032
Date: 13th Septmber 2012

Read: The Transplantation of Human Organs Act, 1994 and the Transplantation of Human Organs Rules, 1995

Government Resolution

1. The successes of organ transplantation and it being the only treatment for end stage organ disease has led to its widespread applicaton. Considering the life saving potential of organ transplantation, the Government is committed to streamlining the procedures for co-ordinating organ transplantation in Marashatra particularly in the light of the current situation of availability of organs for transplantation falling woefully short of the demand. Indeed efficacious donor management and meticulous co-ordination is crucial in maintaining excellent outcomes in organ transplantion.

   There is, at present, no established procedure or guideline to deal with situations that arise when brain deaths occur in hospitals in the state that are not registered under the Transplantation of Human Organs Act, 1994 (THO Act) even when the families of the brain dead persons wish or consent to donate the organs of their deceased family member. It is therefore imperative to permit organs to be retrieved when there is a willingness to donate organs at those centers which have the facilities to maintain brain dead deceased donors, so that more lives of organ failure patients can be saved. Considereing the fact that a large number of brain deaths occur in non-transplant organ retrieval centres. The following orders are issued in the Matter.

2. The Appropriate Authority shall register all hospitals in the State that have an Operation Theatre and Intensive Care Unit (ICU) as Non-Transplant Organ Retrieval Centers (NTORCs). These hospitals are permitted to certify brain death as per the procedures stipulated in the guidelines issued by the Appropriate Authority or Government of Maharashtra and thereafter conduct organ retrieval for therapeutic purposes, but are not permitted to perform actual transplantation of human organs.

3. The procedures stipulated in the guidelines issued by the Appropriate Authority or Government of Maharashtra to be followed by the hospitals registered under Human Organ Transplant Act with the Appropriate Authority, for certifying brain death as per the transplantation of Human Organ Act. with the Appropriate Authority, for certifying brain death as per the Transplantation of Human Organ Act, in those hospitals, will apply for brain death certification in NTORCs as well, in the event of a family of brain dead person consenting to organ donation. If neurosurgeon/neurophysician is not available in the NTORCs then they can utilize the services of neurosurgeon/neurophysician from the Brain Stem death Committee of the Hospital registered under Human Organ Transplant Act by the Appropriate Authority.

4. Any NTORCs can take assistance and support from any hospital registered with the Appropriate Authority as Transplant Center for maintaining the brain dead person in stable condition until organ retrieval is carried out.

5. Whenever a brain death occurs in an NTORC and the deceased person's family consents to organ donation, the NTORC shall contact the Zonal Transplant Co-ordination Committee for Organ allocation as per norms.

6. The organs shall be allocated following the prioritization norms as established by Appropriate Authority for Zonal Transplant Co-ordination committee in the State.

7. All other procedures for cadaveric organ donation and organ retrieval as specified in the Transplantation of Human Organs Act and Rules and other relevant Government orders would apply to NTORCs as well.

By order and in the name of Governor

13.9.2012

(T.C. Benjamin)
Additional Chief Secretary

Annexure

Registered Hospital for Heart Under THOA

Sr. No.	Name of the Hospitals
1	Jaslok Hospital, 15, Dr. G. Deshmukh Marg, Mumbai-400025
2	P.D. Hinduja Hospital, Veer Savarkar Marg, Mahim, Mumbai-400016
3	Asian Heart Institute, G/N Blcok, Bandra Kurla Complex, Bandra (East), Mumbai- 400051
4	Fortis Hospital Ltd., Mulund, Mumbai- 400 078
5	Military Hospital Cardio Thorasic Center, Pune
6	Jupiter Hospital, Thane
7	Kokilaben Dhirubai Ambani and Medical Research Institute, Aachutrao Patwardhan Marg, Four bunglows, Andheri (West), Mumbai - 400 053
8	United CIIGMA Hospital, Aurangabad
9	Ruby Hall Clinic Pune
10	Kamalnayan Bajaj Hospital Gut No. 43, Beed Bypass Road, Bajaj Marg, Satara Parisar, Aurangabad
11	Global Hospital—Super Speciality & Transplant Center, Parel, Mumbai.
12	H.N. Reliance Hospital, Mumbai
13	Six Sigma Medicare & Research Centre, Nashik
14	New Era Hospital Nagpur, Telephone Exchange Chowk, Central Avenue Rd. Nagpur
15	Chopda Medicare & Research Centre's Magnum Heart Institute, College Rd., Nashik
16	Apollo Hospital, Navi Mumbai

Registered Hospital for Lungs Under THOA

Sr. No.	Name of the Hospitals
1	Jaslok Hospital, 15, Dr. G. Deshmukh Marg, Mumbai-400025
2	Military Hospital Cardio Thorasic Center, Pune
3	Jupiter Hospital, Thane
4	Kokilaben Dhirubai Ambani and Medical Research Institute, Aachutrao Patwardhan Marg, Four bunglows, Andheri (West), Mumbai-400 053
5	Fortis Hospital Ltd., Mulund, Mumbai-400 078
6	Ruby Hall Clinic, 40 Sassoon Road, Pune-411001
7	Apollo Hospital, Navi Mumbai

Registered Hospital for Heart and Lungs Under THOA

Sr. No.	Name of the Hospitals
1	Military Hospital Cardio Thorasic Center, Pune
2	Jupiter Hospital, Thane
3	Kokilaben Dhirubai Ambani and Medical Research Institute, Aachutrao Patwardhan Marg, Four bunglows, Andheri (West), Mumbai - 400 053

Registered Hospital for Heart and Lungs Under THOA

Sr. No.	Name of the Hospitals
4	Fortis Hospital Ltd., Mulund, Mumbai- 400 078
5	Ruby Hall Clinic, 40 Sassoon Road, Pune-411001
6	Apollo Hospital, Navi Mumbai

Registered Hospital for Pancreas Under THOA

Sr. No.	Name of the Hospitals
1	KEM Hospital 489, Rastra Peth, Sardar Mudliyar Road, Pune - 411 011.
2	Deenanath Mangeshkar Hospital & Research Center, Erandawane, Pune.
3	Global Hospitals, Parel Mumbai
4	Fortis Hospitals Ltd. Mulund, Mumbai.
5	Ruby Hall Clinic, 40 Sassoon Road, Pune-411001
6	Wockhardt Hospital Ltd., The Umrao Institute of Medical Science and Research, Near Rly Station, Mira Road (E) Thane
7	Wockhardt Hospital Ltd., Mumbai Central
8	Jupiter Hospital Thane

Registered Hospital for Intestine Under THOA

Sr. No.	Name of the Hospitals
1	Global Hospitals, Parel Mumbai
2	Wockhardt Hospital Ltd., Mumbai Central

Registered Hospital for Pancreas and Intestine Under THOA

Sr. No.	Name of the Hospital
1	Global Hospitals, Parel Mumbai

Registered Hospital for Tissue Under THOA

Sr. No.	Name of the Hospitals
1	Tata Memorial Hospital, Mumbai
2	Masina Hospital, Byculla Mumbai
3	National Burn Centre Airoli, Navi Mumbai

Registered Hospital for Pancreas and Kidney Under THOA

Sr. No.	Name of the Hospitals
1	Fortis Hospitals Ltd. Mulund, Mumbai.

Registered Hospital for Hand Transplant Under THOA

Sr. No.	Name of the Hospitals
1	K.E.M Hospital, Parel Mumbai
2	Global Hospital, Parel Mumbai
3	Command Hospital, Pune

Registered Hospital for Uterus Transplant Under THOA

Sr. No.	Name of the Hospitals
1	Galaxy Care Laparoscopy Institute Near Garware College, Ayurvedic Ras-Shala Complex, 25-A, Karve Road, Pune-411004.

List of the Trusts Which Provide Financial Help to the Patients

Mr. Shambhu Dalvi, Community Develpoment Officer, K.E.M. Hospital, Mumbai

Sr. No.	Trust Name	Specification
1	A.H. Wadia Ch. Trust, 70, V.B. Gandhi Marge, Forbs Street Fort, Mumbai	–
2	Aashida Bhau Kulkarni Trust, Ashida Electronic Vagale Estate, Plot no 308, Road No 21 Thane.	–
3	Abu Charitable Trust, 450, Kkatha Bazar, Masjit Bunder (W), Mumbai-400009	–
4	AL Hamad Hospital & Medical, Research Foundation, 55/55A Eleven Star Apartment, Morland Road, Opp. Alana Hall Mumbai-400008	–
5	Allana Foundation, Allana House, Allana Road Opp. Electric House, Colaba, Mumbai-400001.	–
6	Anand Smruti Charitable Trust, 139-A, Ramnivas, Agar Bazar, Dadar (W), Mumbai-400028.	–
7	Basilica of Our Lady of the Mount, Bandra West, Mumbai-400050.	–
8	Being Human, the Salman Khan Foundation, 3, Galaxy pt. B.J. Road. Bandra (W) Bandstand 400050	–
9	Bhairao Charitable Trust, Khadak Road, Shivaji Chowk, Bhiwandi-421302	–
10	Bombay Heart Institute, 516/ Reva Chamners, 5th Floor, 31 Navi Marine Lines, Mumbai-400020.	–
11	Bombay Medical Aid Foundation, Birla Matudhree Sabhagruh Bldg., 1st Floor, OPD Room No. 5,12, New Marine Line, Mumbai-400020	–
12	Bosilica of our lady of the Mound, Bandra, Mumbai-400050	–
13	Budhrani Charitable Trust, 2, Bhadus Court, 1st Pasta Lane, Colaba, Mumbai-400005	–
14	Century Seva Trust, Century Bazar Worli, Mumbai-400025	–
15	Dr. & Mrs. SHM Modi Harmuse House, Benevolence Trust Fund, 2, Arcadia, NCPA Road, Nariman Point, Mumbai-400021	–
16	Dr. Wishawas puranik, Gr. Floor, Opp. To More Store Dombiwali (W) Thane.	–
17	EKAM Foundation, VI House, Ground Floor, Old Prabhadevi, Dadar Mumbai-400025.	Below 18 yrs old Patient
18	Goodlass Nerrolac Paints Ltd. (Trust) Nerolac House, A.G. Kadam Marg, Lower Parel Mumabi-400013	–
19	Gosumec Alummi Association, Gr. Floor, College Bldg, Opp., Dean's Office, Seth G.S. Medical College & K.E.M. Hospital, Parel, Mumbai-400012.	–
20	Haji Ali Dargah trust, Dargah Rd, Haji Ali, Mumbai	–
21	Hon. Chief Minister, Chief Minister Relief Fund, 7th Floor, Mantralaya, Mumbai.	Government Office
22	Hon. Mayor of Mumbai, Mayor's Relief Fund, Mahanagarpalika Office.	Government Office
23	Hon. Prime Minister of India, Prime Minister Relief Fund, New Delhi- 110011.	Government Office
24	Human Welfare Foundation, 513, Commerce house, 140, N.M. Road, Fort, Mumbai-23	–
25	Jai Ganesh Charitable Trust, Bhaivar Export, 94/96, First Floor, Bhagwan Kala Building, Bhuleshwar Road, Mumbai-400002.	–
26	KARO, 414, Empire Complex Senapati Bapat Marge, Lower Parel Mumbai 400013	–

List of the Trusts Which Provide Financial Help to the Patients

Mr. Shambhu Dalvi, Community Develpoment Officer, K.E.M. Hospital, Mumbai

Sr. No.	Trust Name	Specification
27	Katgara Foundation, Elphinstone Bld, 1st Floor, 10, Ver Nariman Road, Mumbai. 400001.	–
28	Khair-e-Ummat Trust, B. IT Chawl No. 1, Imambada Compound, Imambada Mumbai-400009.	–
29	Khidmat Ch. Trust, 106, Sophiya Zubair Road, Nr. Nagpada Police Station, Nagpada Mumbai-400008	–
30	Lalbaugcha Raja Sarvajanik Ganeshotsava Mandal, Lalbaug, Shri Ganesh Nagar, Sane Gurji Marge, Lalbag Mumbai.	
31	Lok Kalyan Nidhi Trust, 201, Rahkiran, M.G. Road, Kandiwali (W), Mumbai-400067.	–
32	Lotus Trust, 6, Louts House, Next to Liberty, Cinema, New Marie line, Mumbai-400001	–
33	Mahavir Heart Research Centre, Avanti Apartment, Sion, Mumbai-22	–
34	Malharbai Foundation, c/o R.L. Hinduja (Trustee), 23/45-d, Vanus Appartment. Dr. R.G. Thadani Marge, Mumbai-400018.	–
35	Motiben Manial Modi Ch. Trust, 51 Priti Sadan Sadan Sikka Nagar V.P. Road. Mumbai 400004	–
36	Motiben Manilal Medical Ch. Trust, 51, Pristi Sadan, Sicka Nagar, V.P. Road, Mumbai-4	–
37	Nana Palkar Smruti Samittee, 158, Chamarbaug Cross St. Dr Ambedkar Road, Parel, Mumbai-400012.	–
38	Navneet Foundation Lakhanibai Ch. Trust, Navneet Bhavan, Bhawani Shankar Road, Dadar, Mumbai- 400028	–
39	Nirlon Foundation, Nirlon House, 254-B, Dr. Annie Besant Road, Worli, Mumbai-400030	–
40	Phirozshah Godrej Foundation, Godrej Bhavan, N.A. House, Fort, Mumbai-400001	–
41	Pujari Julelal Mandir (Chartiable Trust) Ulhasnagar-5, Dist-Thane.	
42	Rabai Abdul Kedar Millwala Aminchand Mension, D Wing, 16, Maden Cama Road, New Golden Gate Hotle, Regal Cinema, Mumbai- 40008	–
43	Ramlila Charities, Plot 13, Western Industrial Co-op Estate, MIDC Andheri (E), Mumbai-400092.	–
44	Rastrapati Cachivalay, Rastrapati Bhavan, New Delhi-110004.	Government Office
45	Rishikesh Marthallkar, Rotang Club, Nasik, 34, New Rajan Complex, Arcade, Datta Mandir stop, Nasik Road, Nasik-422101	–
46	Shalini Bansal, JSW foundation, pandurang Ibhutkar Road, Victoriya House, 2nd Floor, lower Parel, Mumbai-400013.	–
47	Shree Mahalakshmi Temple Ch. Bhulabhai Dasai Road, Mumbai-400026.	–
48	Shree Siddhivinayak Ganapati Temple Trust, S.K. Bole Marg, Prabhadevi, Mumbai-400028	–
49	Shree Venkteshwar Nidi, Plot No. R-856, TTC Industrial Area, Rabale, Post-Ghansoli, Navi Mumbai-400701	–
50	Shri Nilkantheshwar Temple, Religious Trust, Worli, 126, Nilkantheshwar Bhuvan, 5, Second Floor, Dr. Annie Besent Road, Worli, Mumbai-400018	–

List of the Trusts Which Provide Financial Help to the Patients

Mr. Shambhu Dalvi, Community Develpoment Officer, K.E.M. Hospital, Mumbai

Sr. No.	Trust Name	Specification
51	Shri Saibaba Sandthan, 804 B, 3rd Floor, SAI Niketan Building, Dr. Ambedkar Road, Dadar East, Mumbai-400014.	–
52	Shri Saibaba Sansthan, Shirdhi, Tal. Kopargaon, Dist Ahmednagar.	–
53	Shri. N.M. Wadia Charities, N.M. Wadia Bleg., 123, M.G. Road, Mumbai-400023.	–
54	Sindhu Charitable Society, 132, Katara Mansion Dr. B.A. Road Worli Naka Mumbai 400017	–
55	Sir Ratan Tata Trust, Mulla House, Jehangir Wadoa Blug., 3rd Floor, 51, M.G. Road, Mumbai- 400001	–
56	Smt. Parmila Shantilal Shah Ch,. Foundation, Construction House, 5 Walchand Hiranand Road, Belard Estate, Mumbai-400001.	–
57	St. Michael's Church, L.J. Road, Near Bus Depot, Mahim, Mumbai-400016	–
58	Suman Ramesh Tulsani Ch. Trust, 1103/04, Tulasani Chambers, 212, Nariman Point, Mumbai-400001	–
59	Sushila Modi Charitable Trust, 6/7 Dosa Menson, 1st Floor, Near Apna Bazar, Sir Pm Rd., Fort Mumbai. 400001	–
60	Swami Shanti Prakash Ashram Trust, Ulhasnagar-5, Dist-Thane.	–
61	Taiba Welfare Trust, 126, Kamberkar Street, Mumbai-400003.	–
62	Tata Chem Golden Jubilee Foundation Holland House-2nd Floor, Near Regal Cinema, 14 Shaheed Bhagat Singh Road Colaba Mumbai 400001	–
63	Tata Education and Development Trust, Bombay House, Ground Floor, Homi Mody Street, Fort Mumbai-400001	–
64	Tavescor Charitable Trust, Elphinstone Building, 2nd Floor, 10 Veer Nariman Road, Mumbai-400001	–
65	The Health Officer, Health Dept. Zila Parishad	
66	The Navneet Foundation, Navneet Bhavan, Bhawani Shanker Road, Dadar, Mumbai-400028	–
67	V.M. Modi 51. Priti Station, Sikka Nagar, Sir V.P. Road, Near V.P. Police Station Mumbai-400003.	–

List of the Documents Required for Help from Trust

Sr. No.	Documents
1	Ration Card
2	Income Certificate
3	Doctor's letter with cost estimate
4	Self-Application
5	Photo ID proof
6	Xerox copy of Bank Statement or Passbook
7	Electricity Bill, etc.

Note: Approximate cost of kidney transplant in Govrenment Hospital—5 lakhs including immunosupression for 1 year

Approximate cost of liver transplant in Government Hospital—9 lakhs including immunosupression for 1 year

Approximate cost of kidney transplant in Government Hospital—7–8 lakhs excluding immunosupression

Approximate cost of liver transplant in private Hospital—22 to 25 lakhs

Under Transplantation of Human organs Act 1994 following the status the Centers registered as Non-Transplant organ Retrieved Centre in the State

Sr. No.	Name of the Hospital	Type of Hospital (Govt. /Mun./Pvt.)	No. of Beds	Registration given date
1	Govt. Medical College & Hospital Yeotmal	Govt.	594	01.06.2013
2	RCSM Govt. Med. College & C. P. R. Hospital Kolhapur	Govt.	665	15.06.2013
3	Civil Hospital, Ratnagiri	Govt.	200	09.05.2013
4	Govt. Medical College & Hospital Latur	Govt.	520	27.05.2013
5	Civil Hospital Aundh, Pune	Govt.	300	25.03.2013
6	V. N. Desai Gen. Hosp., Santacruz, Mumbai	Mun.	254	07.04.2013
7	General Hospital, Gondia	Govt.	200	27.08.2013
8	St. George Hosp., Mumbai	Govt.	467	23.01.2013
9	Bhagavati Gen. Hosp., Borivali, Mumbai	Mun.	373	21.04.2013
10	Bhabha Mun. Gen. Hosp., Bandra, Mumbai	Mun.	436	15.04.2013
11	Navi Mumbai Mun. Gen. Hosp., Vashi	Mun.	300	06.04.2013
12	G. T. Hosp., Mumbai	Govt.	521	23.01.2013
13	Yashwantrao Chavan Mun. Gen. Hosp., Pimpri Chinchwad Pune	Mun.	750	30.03.2013
14	M. T. Agarwal Mun. Gen. Hosp., Mulund, Mumbai.	Mun.	225	15.04.2013
15	Rajiv Gandhi Medi. College & CSM Hosp. Kalwa	Mun.	500	16.04.2013
16	Rajawadi Mun. Gen. Hosp., Ghatkokpar, Mumbai	Mun.	580	15.04.2013
17	Siddharth Mun. Gen. Hosp. Goregaon, Mumbai	Mun.	172	28.04.2013
18	General Hospital Sindhudurga	Govt.	100	18.04.2013
19	General Hospital Beed	Govt.	320	25.03.2013
20	General Hospital Thane	Govt.	336	25.03.2013
21	General Hospital Osamanabad	Govt.	236	25.03.2013
22	General Hospital Ulhasnagar	Govt.	202	16.04.2013
23	General Hospital, Chandrapur	Govt.	300	29.04.2013
24	General Hospital, Wardha	Govt.	286	18.04.2013
25	General Hospital, Gadchiroli	Govt.	226	03.05.2013
26	General Hospital, Raigad (Alibaug)	Govt.	272	29.03.2013
27	Civil Hospital, Jalna	Govt.	200	05.12.2013
28	Civil Hospital, Hingoli	Govt.	100	01.01.2014
29	Civil Hospital, Nashik	Govt.	541	28.03.2014
30	Umrao Inst. Of Medical Science & Research Center, Mira Road, Thane	Pvt.	200	16.6.2014
31	Bethani Hospital, Thane	Pvt.	125	11.7.2014
32	Asian Inst. Of Medical Sciences, Dombivali	Pvt.	100	27.7.2014
33	Civil Hospital Bhandara	Govt.	400	26.9.2014
34	Dr. Vasantrao Pawar Medical College & Hospital, Adgaon, Nasik	Pvt.	1000	04.02.2015
35	Sushrut Hospital & Research Center, Mumbai	Trust	67	04.03.2015
36	Cigma Hospital, Aurangabad	Pvt.	52	23.4.2015
37	Dist. Hospital, Ahmednagar	Govt	274	07.07.2015
38	Civil Hospital, Nandurbar	Govt	200	07.07.2015

Sr. No.	Name of the Hospital	Type of Hospital (Govt. /Mun./Pvt.)	No. of Beds	Registration given date
	Under Transplantation of Human organs Act 1994 following the status the Centers registered as Non-Transplant organ Retrieved Centre in the State			
39	Civil Hospital Jalgaon	Govt	356	07.07.2015
40	Noble Hospital & Research Center, Ahmednagar	Trust	113	17.07.2015
41	Dr. Shankar Rao Chavan Govt. Medi. Col., Nanded	Govt	508	17.07.2015
42	Rao Nursing Home Pune	Pvt	123	24.7.2015
43	Dist. Hospital Buldhana	Govt	306	17.10.2015
44	Dist. Hospital Amaravati	Govt	379	17.10.2015
45	Civil Hosp., Washim	Govt	100	17.10.2015
46	Govt. Med. College Akola	Govt	554	06.11.2015
47	Govt. Med. College Solapur	Govt	800	02.12.2015
48	Surya Sahyadri Hospital Pune	Pvt.	75	7/1/2016
49	Nirmaya Hospital Chinchgaon Pune	Pvt.	110	11/1/2016
50	Govt. Medical College Aurangabad	Govt	1170	02.01.2016
51	Smt. Kashibai Navale Med. College & Hospital Pune	Pvt.	934	05/03/2016
52	Shri Bhausaheb Sardeshai Medical college Pune	Pvt.	665	18/03/2016
53	Govt. Medical College Ambajogai Dist. Beed	Govt.	518	28/04/2016
54	Govt. Medical College Miraj Dist. Sangli	Govt.	320	04/06/2016
55	Govt. Medical College Chandrapur	Govt.	600	15/02/2017
56	Gangamai Hospital, Solapur	Pvt.	100	09/05/2017

ORGAN AND DISTRIBUTION IN BRAIN STEM DEAD (BSD) DONORS

Step 1: Informing the Zonal Transplant Coordination Cenre (ZTCC) Coordinator

After the first apnoea test, if the family is willing to donate organs, call the ZTCC coordinator to inform him/her about a potential donor and the organs for which consent for donation has been obtained.

Provide the following details to the ZTCC Coordinator:

1. Donor Medical History
2. Medicolegal case or non-medicolegal case
3. Tentative retrieval time
4. Body handover timing (If family has specificed a timing)

Step 2: Informing Organ Committee Chairperson

After getting the details mentioned in step 1 the ZTCC coordinator needs to inform the organ committees' chairpersons about the potential donor with medical details, and ask for their expert opinion for eligibility of the donor.

The ZTCC coordinator also needs to inform the technician who performs the crossmatching tests in the case of kidney, heart and lung donation.

Step 3: Distribution of Organs

In the case of a multi-organ donor in a registered transplant centre, if there are suitable recipients, all organs may be utilised by the donor hospital as per the hospital waiting list, except for one kidney which shall be allocated as per the ZTCC waiting list.

In the case of a multi-organ donor in a registered non-transplant organ retrieval centre (NTORC) all organs shall be allocated as per the ZTCC waiting list.

Distribution of organs will be done as detailed below.

A. KIDNEY DISTRIBUTION

The patient waiting list for kidney goes as per the score and donor age.

The ZTCC Co-ordinator has to maintain the waiting list. They are also responsible for assigning the score as per the criteria given in the ZTCC/SOTTO Guidelines.

Age groups are maintained as follows:

Age 3–5 years = Age group 1

Age 5–10 years = Age group 2

Age 11–45 years = Age group 3

Age above 45 years = Age group 4

Recipients of the same age group as the donor are allotted two extra points and distribution done accordingly.

The ZTCC coordinator should have the above list for distribution.

One Kidney is allocated to the donor hospital and the second kidney is allocated as per the city waiting list. If there are no recipients in the city list then the kidney is offered to the State through the State Organ and Tissue Transplant Organisation (SOTTO), then to other States in the Region through the Regional Organ and Tissue Transplant Organisation (ROTTO) and finally to other States through National Organ and Tissue Transplant Organisation NOTTO.

For every kidney donation the blood of 2 to 3 patients are sent for crossmatching, from the city waiting list as well as from hospital waiting list

B. LIVER DISTRIBUTION

The patient waiting list for liver is maintained according to chronology. For liver distribution the priority is as follows:
  1. Super urgent waitlisted patient
  2. Donor hospital waitlisted patient
  3. City waitlisted patient (If the donor hospital does not have a suitable patient.)

During distribution three patients are counselled and clinically prepared, one for transplant and the other two as standby. Blood is sent for crossmatching.

If there are no recipients in the city list then the liver is offered to the State through SOTTO, then to other States in the Region through ROTTO and finally to other States through NOTTO.

If a hospital refuses a liver during retrieval on medical grounds then it is the responsibility of the hospital's retrieval team to conduct an on table frozen section biopsy to check if the liver is medically suitable for transplant or not, and submit the results to ZTCC.

C. HEART DISTRIBUTION

The patient waiting list for heart is maintained according to chronology. For heart distribution the priority is as follows:
  1. Super urgent waitlisted patient
  2. Donor hospital waitlisted patient
  3. City waitlisted patient (If donor hospital does not have a suitable patient.)

During distribution three patients are prepared, one for transplant and the other two as standby. Blood is sent for crossmatching.

If there are no recipients in the city list then the heart is offered to the State through SOTTO, then to other States in the Region through ROTTO and finally to other States through NOTTO.

D. PERSONS TO BE INFORMED

During the distribution of organs the ZTCC coordinator needs to inform the following:
  1. Crossmatch technician: List of patients who will be coming for crossmatch.
  2. Donor hospital: List of the hospitals where organs are allocated for further retrieval coordination.
  3. Donor hospital and recipient hospital: Crossmatch report.
  4. Executive members of ZTCC and ROTTO: After final distribution.

Transplant coordinator list Mumbai				
	Hospitals	*Hospital address*	*Transplant Coordinator name*	*Official mobile nos.*	*Email ID*
1.	Apollo Hospital	Plot no.13, Parsik Hill road, Off Uran road, CBD Belapur, opp. New wonders park, Navi Mumbai-400614	Prakash Saindane	8108993820 / 96198 94281	transplant_nm@apollohospitals.com
2.	Asian Heart Instt.	G/N Block, Bandra-Kurla Complex, Bandra(E), Mumbai-400051, India	Prashant K Jadhav	9975002491	mrd@ahirc.com / transplant.coordinator@ahirc.com
3.	Bombay Hospital	12, New Marine lines, Mumbai 400 020	Rajendra Khairmode	7021853121	
4.	Bhaktivedanta Hospital	Mira Road	Dr. Apeksha Kanchan	7506094996	transplant@bhaktivedantahospital.com/ drapeksha.kanchan@ bhaktivedantahospital.com
5.	Breach Candy Hosp.	Haji Ali	Dr. Kavitha Shah	8879033711 / 9930234969/ 9820713069	drkavita@breachcandyhospital.org
6.	Criticare Hospital	Andheri	Sameer More	9594555569	transplant@criticarehospital.in
7.	D.Y. Patil	Nerul	Nitin Yeshwante	9967105040	ns.1760@rediffmail.com
8.	Fortis Hospitals Ltd., Mulund	Mulund Goregaon link road, Mulund (west), Mumbai 400078	Nishant Sarvagod/ Vijetha Shetty/ Sudarshan Bhoir	9220862659/ 9892266809/ 9082311755/ 8655302425	nishant.sarvagod@fortishealthcare.com/ vijeetha.shetty@fortishealthcare.com
9.	Fortis-Hiranandani Hospital	Plot No: 28, Sector: 10A, Mini Seashore Road, Vashi, Navi Mumbai-400703	Madonna Hynniewta	9152855488	Organdonation.vashi@fortishealthcare.com
10.	Global Hospital	Parel	Ms. Disha Jadhav	82910 47210	msw@globalhospitalsindia.com
11.	Godrej Hospital	Pirojsha Nagar, Eastern Express Highway, Vikhroli-east, Mumbai 400079	Mr. Ramzan Khalif	9619894284	hospital@godrej.com
12.	H.N. Reliance Foundation Hosp	Charni Road	Mr. Praful Nawar	9930 255625	Praful.nawar@rfhospital.org
13.	P.D. Hinduja Hospital	Dadar, Shivaji Park	Mr. Santosh Sorate	9850852502	
14.	Hira-Mongi Navneet Hosp	Mulund	Dr. Janhavi	9821181810	shreepragatifoundation@yahoo.co.in
15.	INHS Hospital	Colaba	Ms. Laxmi Tole	8433598778	tolelaxmi853@gmail.com
16.	J. J. Hospital	Byculla	Premsingh Rathod/Sunil Patil	8356971581/ 9029257895/ 8806862739	sunilpatil6899@yahoo.com/ premsinghrathod369@gmail.com
17.	Jaslok Hosp.	15, Dr. G. Deshmukh Marg, Pedder road, Mumbai-400 026	Ramakant Dhas	9702260837	msw@jaslokhospital.net/ www.jaslokhospital.net

Transplant coordinator list Mumbai

	Hospitals	Hospital address	Transplant Coordinator name	Official mobile nos.	Email ID
18.	Jupiter Hospital	Jupiter Lifeline Hospital Ltd. Eastern Express Highway, Thane (w) 400601	Anirudh Kulkarni	9757303463/ 9869544210	anirudha.kulkarni@jupiterhospital.com
19.	Kohinoor Hospital	Kohinoor City, Kirol Road, Off LBS Marg, Kurla West, Mumbai 400070, India	Manisha Rankhambe	9320493839	manisha.rankhambe@kohinoorhospitals.in www.kohinoorhospitals.in
20.	Kokilaben D. Ambani Hosp	Andheri (W), Mumbai-400053	Rekha Barot/ Abhijeet Sinker	9321163693 9769428097 9321801408	rekha.barot@relianceada.com / abhijeet.sinkar@relianceada.com
21.	KEM Hosp.	Parel	Dr. Abhinav Katyal (kidney)	9860316074/ 9766744697	drharrison4u@gmail.com
22.	Lilavati Hospital	A-791, Bandra Reclamation, Bandra (west), Mumbai - 400 050	Mr. Pramod Shinge	9769840408 / 9960955453	sewa@lilavatihospital.com
23.	L.T.M.G. Hospital	Sion west	Dr. Amandeep Arora	9833739090	amamarora12389@gmail.com
24.	M.G.M Hospital-Kamothe (New Bombay Hospital)	Panvel,	Yogesh Sakhare/ Vaishali Aher/ Rupali Gujar/ Bagul	8108174464/ 9702903483/ 8369476323/ 9321441777	
25.	M.G.M Hospital-Vashi	Vashi, Navi Mumbai 400 703	Vaibhav Bhosle	9870057514	vashimgm@gmail.com / vaibhav275@gmail.com
26.	Mallika Hospital		Dr. Bhupendra	9819419256	hospital.m@gmail.com
27.	Nanavati Hospital	Vile Parle	Rahul Wasnik/ Anand Sirsath.	9619110098/ 9702084689/ 9421383372	transplantcoordinator@ nanavatihospital.org/ rajendra.patankar@nanavatihospital.org
28.	Nair Hosp.	Bombay Central	Dr. Kalpana Mehata/Jaya Saket	9322226090/ 8793714123	jsakat2009@gmail.com
29.	Prince Aly Khan Hosp.	Mazgaon	Nitin Tambe	9172490558	transplant@pakh.net
30.	Parakh Hospital	Ghatkopar East	Dr. Meena Dani-Dialysis unit/ Aditya Sahu	9320605750	parakhhospital@gmail.com
31.	S.L. Raheja Hosp.	Raheja Rugnalaya Marg, Mahim (west) Mumbai-400	Sachin Savle	9004479512/ 9167111938	transplant.coordinator@rahejahospital.com
32.	Seven Hills Hospitals	Andheri East			
33.	Saifee Hospital	Charni road	Dr. Shabina/ Mona	9223290636, 9403660906/ 9833444905	write@saifeehospital.in
34.	Wockhardt Hospital-Mumbai Central	Dr. Anand Rao Nair Road, South Mumbai, Mumbai- 400 011	Bhavana Shah	7506030195/ 7506655509	Bhavana.Shah@wockhardthospitals.com/ transplant@wockhardthospitals.com
35.	Umrao Wockhardt-	Mira Road	Amol Kadam	7387156659	Transplant.Nobo@wockhardthospitals.com

No.	Name of the coordinator/hospital	Contact no.	Email ID
	Transplant coordinator list Pune		
1	**Vaishali Phansalkar** Poona Hospital **Address:** 27, Sadashiv Peth, Nr. Alka Talkies, Pune, Maharashtra 411030	9158922264	vaishali.a.phansalkar@gmail.com
2	**Shilpa Barve** Deenanath Mangeshkar Hosp. **Address:** Near Mhatre Bridge, Pune, Maharashtra 411004	9850953534	transplant.cd@dmhospital.org shilpbarve@gmail.com
3	**Surekha Joshi** Ruby Hall Clinic **Address:** 40, Sassoon Road, Sangamvadi, Pune, Maharashtra 41100	9975303002	mswoffice@rubyhall.com
4	**Rohini Shahastrabuddhe** KEM Hospital **Address:** 489, Sardar Moodliar Road, Rasta Peth, Pune, Maharashtra 411011	9823505327	rodie27feb@gmail.com
5	**Sagar Kakkad** Jupiter Hospital **Address:** Mahatma Jyotiba Phule Bridge, Near Prathamesh Park Road, Baner, Pune, Maharashtra 411045	9011016124	SAGARKAKAD16@hotmail.com
6	**Rahul Tambe (Liver Coordinator)** SSH Deccan Gym. **Address:** Plot No. 30-C, Erandvane, Karve Rd, Deccan Gymkhana, Pune, Maharashtra 411004	9923674260	rahul.tambe@sahyadrihospitals.com rahul.tambe@sahyadrihospitals.com
7	**Sharmila Padhye** SSH Deccan Gym **Address:** Plot No. 30-C, Erandvane, Karve Rd, Deccan Gymkhana, Pune, Maharashtra 411004	9850873274	socialworker@sahyadrihospitals.com
8	**Nitin Dushing** SSH Ngr, Rd	9673355448	transplant.ngr@sahyadrihospitals.com
9	**Bobin Methew** Birla Hospital **Address:** Aditya Birla Marg, Thergaon, Pimpri-Chinchwad, Maharashtra 411033	7030482451	abmh-pune.msw@adityabirla.com
10	**Prkash Nimbore** Budhrani Hospital **Address:** 7–9, 1st Ln, Vasani Nagar, Koregaon Park, Pune, Maharashtra 411001	9850224042	inlaksbb@gmail.com
11	**Vrunda Pusalkar** Jehangir Hospital **Address:** 32, Sasoon Road, Opposite Railway Station, Central Excise Colony, Sangamvadi, Pune, Maharashtra 411001	8888821088	vrinda.pusalkar@jehangirhospital.com

No.	Name of the coordinator/ hospital	Contact no.	Email ID
	Transplant coordinator list Pune		
12	**Rucha Borwankar** Inamdar Hospital **Address:** Buildings, Inamdar Hospital, No. 15, Fatima Nagar, Pune, Maharashtra 411040	9011000201	borwankarrucha@gmail.com
13	**Arjun Rathod** BJMC & Sasoon Gen. Hospital **Address:** Agarkar Nagar, Jai Prakash Narayan Road, Near Pune Railway Station, Pune, Maharashtra 411001	9404676873	arjun.rathod1@gmail.com
14	**Vishal Torde** Nobel Hospital **Address:** 153, Magarpatta City Road, Hadapsar, Pune, Maharashtra 411013	7875443351	vishalbird@gmail.com
15	**Amol Dujage** Wockhardt Hospital **Address:** Wani House, Mumbai - Agra Highway, Wadala Naka, Nashik, Maharashtra 422001	8600959444	Amol.Dugaje@wockhardthospitals.com
16	**Charusheela Jadhav** Apollo Hospital **Address:** Plot No. 1, Swaminarayan Nagar, New Adgaon Naka, Panchavati, Near Lunge Mangal Karyalaya, Nashik, Maharashtra 422003	9270382355	charusheela_j@apollohospitals.com
17	**Mahesh Benkudale** Saibaba Heart Inst. & Research Centre **Address:** Near Kalidas Kala Mandir, Shalimar, Nashik, Maharashtra 422001	8485843208	saibabaheartinstitute@yahoo.com
18	**Dr. Sanjay Rakibe** Rishikesh Hospital **Address:** 9 Gangapur Rd, Murkute Colony, Nashik, Maharashtra 422002	9960125555	sanjayrakibe@gmail.com
19	**Poonam** Six Sigma Hospital **Address:** Satguru's, Opp Water Tank, Mahatma Nagar, Nashik, Maharashtra 422007	9762738063	
20	**Kavita Rahatwal** Apple Hospital **Address:** 804/2, 805/2, E Ward, Circuit House To Kadamwadi Road, Bhosalewadi, Kolhapur, Maharashtra 416003	7770003584	rhatwalkavita10@gmail.com
21	**Swarupakawalgi** Ashvini Sahakri Hospital **Address:** North Sadar Bazaar, Solapur, Maharashtra 413003	8625806689	swashree21@gmail.com

No.	Name of the coordinator/ hospital	Contact no.	Email ID
	Transplant coordinator list Pune		
22	**Dr. Anand Salgar** Diamond super S. hospital **Address:** Bawada Road, Next To Mahaveer College, Ramanmala, Kolhapur, Maharashtra 416003	8856910510	diamondhospitalkop@gmail.com
23	**Sukant Bele** Yashodhara Super speciality Hospital **Address:** Sidheshwar Peth, Solapur, Maharashtra 413001	8888627176	sukantbele@gmail.com
24	**Vaishali Yadav** Krishna Hospital **Address:** Khanapur Road, Agashivnagar, District Satara, Malkapur, Maharashtra 415539	8390730994	
25	**Dr. Aniket Suryawanshi** Aster Adhar Hospital **Address:** R. S. No. 628, 'B' Ward, Near Shastri Nagar, Near KMT Workshop, Kolhapur, Maharashtra 416012	9225256009	aniket.suryawanshi@asteraadhar.com
26	**Mayuri Ghadage** D Y Patil Hospital **Address:** Dr. D. Y. Patil Medical College, Hospital & Research Centre, Sant Tukaram Nagar, Pimpri Colony, Pune, Maharashtra 411018	9850975314	mayurighadage@gmail.com transplant.coordinator@dpu.edu.in
27	**Sham Borale** Shree Vighnharta Hospital – 21 Abhushan, Old Chiranrar Hospital Rana Pratap Colony, Depur, Dhule 424001	7875975110	svh.dhule@gmail.com
28	**Dr. Sandeep Holkar** ARMCH– **Address:** At Post. Kumbhari, Tal. South Solapur, Solapur, Maharashtra 413006		drsandeep.holkar@gmail.com
29	**Jasmeet Kaur (Liver Coordinator)** KEM Hospital **Address:** 489, Sardar Moodliar Road, Rasta Peth, Pune, Maharashtra 411011	8698650334	livertransplant@kemhospital.org
30	**Prashant Kulkarni (Liver Coordinator)** Deenanath Mangeshkar Hosp.– **Address:** Near Mhatre Bridge, Pune, Maharashtra 411004	7972503802	liver.tc@dmhospital.org
31	**Aman Bele** SSH Nasik	9028667433	
32	**Dr. Swati Nikam (Heart Tx Coordinator)** Sahyadri Hospital , Deccan Gym.	9881454040	heartrevival@sahyadrihospitals.com

Transplant coordinator list Aurangabad

Sr. No.	Transplant coordinator name	Hospital	Email ID and contact number
1	Mr. Manoj Gadekar	MGM Medical College & Hospital Aurangabad	9975704874 transplantcoordinatormgm@gmail.com
2	Mr. Amol Mudliyar	Kamalnayan Bajaj Hospital Aurangabad	8888958465 transplantcoordinator@bajajhospital.com
3	Mr. Sandip Chavan	United Ciigma Hospital Aurangabad	9158608666 sandipchavan590@gmail.com
4	Mr. Jitendra Kurkure	Manik Hospital & Research Center Aurangabad	9309915997 jitendrakurkure1989@gmail.com
5	Mrs. Lajwanti Dande	Seth Nandalal Dhoot Hospital Aurangabad	9822803583l ajwantidande@gmail.com
6	Mr. Shankar Pote	Sunrise Global Superspeciality Hospital Nanded	7709818736 Shankarpote13795@gmail.com

ZTCC–Nagpur Zone: Transplant coordinators list

Sr. No.	Name	Hospital name	Contact no.	Email ID
1	Dr ved Sarangpure	Meditrina institute of Medical science nagpur	9301122849	vedsarang10@gmail.com
2	Dr Bhavana Methwani	Wochardt Hospital, Nagpur	9511785594	bhavana.methwani@wockhardthospitals.com
3	Dr. Ashwini choudhary	New era Hospital Nagpur	9011792011	ashwini.choudhary79@gmail.com
4	Shubhangi Pokale	Care Hospitals, Nagpur.	9370286116	shubhangi.pokale@carehospitals.com
5	Dr. Mehraj Sheika	Government Superspeciality hospital	9552462248	goldenmeraj28@gmail.com
6	Dr.Sandeep m. Nagmote	Sevenstar Hospital	9158441525	dr.sandeepnagmote@gmail.com
7	Dr Ashish Anwikar	Meditrina Institute of Medical Sciences	9226571846	ashishanwikar@gmail.com
8	Mrs. Manjiri Damle	Oragne City Hospital & Research Institiute	9763412153	manjiridamle@live.com
9	Mrs. Veena Wathore	ZTCC-Nagpur	9112298235	veenawathore@gmail.com
10	Kanchan Shewde	Meditrina Institute of Medical Sciences.	7620632711/ 9372760691	kanchanshewde@gmail.com
11	Bulu Behera	Mohan Foundation— Nagpur	9595275920/ 7387023971	bulu@mohanfoundation.org
12	Shyam Panjala	GMCH, Nagpur	9689881100	shyam.panjala12@gmail.com
13	Preety Jain	Alexis Hospital	8788924439	pgjain@alexishospital.com
14	Mrunali khonde	Alexis Hospital	7030923413/ 9850927547	mkhonde@alexishospital.com
15	Rupali Naik	Acharya Vinoba Bhave Rural Hospital, Wardha	9579172011	naikrupali23@rediffmail.com
16	Dr. Hema Dhoble	Sure Tech Hospital, Nagpur	9890188853	drhemadhoble@gmail.com

विशेष पोलीस पत्रक

विशेष पोलीस परिपत्रक परिच्छेद क्रमांक ४५/२००९, दिनांक २८.१०.२००९

सह पोलीस आयुक्त (एन्.), मुंबई

परिपत्रक
दि. २७.१०.२००९

विषय : Zonal Transplant Co-ordination Centre या संस्थेस सहकार्य करणेबाबत.

काही विधिवैद्यकीय (Medico Legal Cases) प्रकरणांमध्ये अखनी अथवा अंतरूग्ण वलीत व्यक्ती जेव्हा मृत्युशय्येवर असते, त्यावेळी त्याचे रक्ताचे नातेवाईक (Blood Relatives) यांना जखमी/अंतरूग्ण व्यक्तीचे अवयव दान करण्याबाबत निर्णय घेतात. असे अवयव दान करतात. ऐते व्यक्तीच्या मृत्युनंतर तात्काळ ते अवयव मृत शरीरापासून वमळ करून उपलोहित आपलीले करतात. त्यामुळे अशा प्रकरणांमध्ये भेसूबीज संबंधेकडून अनावश्यक विलंब न होणे अपेक्षित आहेत.

याबाबतचे काम Zonal Transplant Co-ordination Centre लोकमान्य टिळक रूग्णालय, सायन, मुंबई ही करत असल्याने दाखल एडने. तरी यांद्रे वरी निर्देशित करण्यात आले की अशा प्रकरणांमधील इसमाच्या मृत्युची खबर पोलीस ठाण्यास मिळताच संबंधित पोलीस अधिकारी खालील प्रमाणे दक्षता घ्यावी.

१) वर्तमानातील अशी अंमलदाराने प्रथम रोगीणार्गे तथा रूग्णालयात जावून पूर्वराहाच्या तात्काळ फौ.द.प्र.सं. कलम १७४ अन्वये इन्क्वेस्ट पंचनामा करावा.

२) अशा प्रकरणांमधील अपमृत्यु (A.D.R.) नोंदीबाबतची आवश्यक ती कागदपत्रे उदा. एकजाण, जबाब व इन्क्वेस्ट फॉर्म इत्यादी विनाविलंब भराण करावेत व मृत इसमाच्या नातेवाईकांची कोणतीही गैरसोय होणार नाही दक्षता घ्यावी.

३) उपरोक्त Zonal Centre च्या प्रतिनिधींना योग्य ते सहकार्य करावे.

पोलीस आयुक्त, मुंबई

POLICE NOC FORMAT

प्रती,   दिनांक -

मा. वैद्यकीय अधिकारी

————————— हॉस्पीटल

—————————

विषय ः **अवयव दान करिण्या करीता ना हरकत प्रमाणपत्र**

संदर्भ ः हॉस्पीटलचे पत्र दि. ———————

उपरोक्त विषय व संदर्भास अनुसरून कळविण्यात येते की,
आपण सदर पत्राव्दारे श्री/श्रीमती. ——————————— यांचे मस्तिष्क
स्तंभ मृत स्थितीत (Brain Death) अवयव दान करिण्या करीता नाहरकत प्रमाणपत्र
मागितले आहे.

त्यास अनुसरून मेंदू मृत श्री/श्रीमती. ———————————
यांचे वारस व नातेवाईक यांच्या इच्छेनूसार सदर मेंदू मृत (Brain Dead) असलेल्या
इसमाचे ——————————— या अवयवांचे दान करिण्याकरीता
त्यांनी सहमती दिलेली आहे.

या अनुषंगाने सदर इसम श्री/श्रीमती. ———————————
यांचे वारस व नातेवाईक यांची चौकशी करिता त्यांनी सहमती दर्शविलेली आहे.

तरी सदर मेंदू मृत (Brain Dead) इसम श्री/श्रीमती. ——————— यांचे
अवयव दान करण्याबाबत पोलिसांची काहीही हरकत नाही.

कळावे,

पोलिस ठाणे अंमलदार

————— पोलिस ठाणे

FORMAT FOR LETTER FROM HOSPITAL TO POLICE

Date

To,

The Police Sub Inspector/In–charge,

.... Police Station,

....

....

Respected Sir,

Mr./Ms./Master .... is case of brain stem death/death admitted to .... Hospital on date ....
It is the Medico legal case ADR No. ....
As per organ Transplant Act 1994 , the relatives have given consent to donate his/her following organs ....

We request you to give No objection certificate for retrieval. We also request to visit the hospital for the same.

Please, do the needful,

Thanking you,

Medical officer,

.... Hospital

FORMS AS PER THOT RULES, 2014

FORM 1
FOR ORGAN OR TISSUE DONATION FROM IDENTIFIED LIVING NEAR RELATED DONOR
(To be completed by him or her)
(Refer rules 3 and 5(3)(a))

My full name (proposed donor) is ....
and this is my photograph.

Photograph of the Donor
(Attested by Notary Public
across the photo after affixing)

To be affixed here.

My permanent home address is ....
.... Tel: ....
My present address for correspondence is...
.... Tel:....................
Date of birth .... (Day/month/year)

I enclose copies of the following documents: (attach attested photocopy of at least two of following relevant documents to indicate your near relationship):
- Ration/Consumer Card number and Date of issue and place: .... and/or
- Voter's I-Card number, date of issue, Assembly constituency.. and/or
- Passport number and country of issue.. and/or
- Driving License number, Date of issue, licensing authority.. and/or
- Permanent Account Number (PAN)... and/or
- AADHAAR No. .... and/or
- Any other valid proof of identity and address reflecting near relationship ....

I authorize removal for therapeutic purposes and consent to donate my .... (Name of organ/tissue) to my relative .... (Specify son/daughter/father/mother/brother/sister/grandfather/grand-mother/grand-son/grand-daughter), whose particulars are as follows and name is .... and who was born on .... (day/month/month):

Photograph of the Recipient
(Attested by Notary Public
across the photo after affixing)

To be affixed here.

The copies of following documents of recipient are enclosed (attach attested photocopy of at least two relevant documents to indicate your near relationship):
- Ration/Consumer Card number and Date of issue and place: .... and/or
- Voter's I-Card number, date of issue, Assembly constituency .... and/or
- Passport number and country of issue .... and/or
- Driving License number, Date of issue, licensing authority .... and/or
- Permanent Account Number (PAN) .... and/or

- AADHAAR No (Issued by Unique Identification Authority of India) ……………………..…………….. and/or
- Any other valid proof of identity and address reflecting near relationship …....…………………………..

I solemnly affirm and declare that:

Sections 2, 9 and 19 of The Transplantation of Human Organs Act, 1994 have been explained to me and I confirm that:

1. I understand the nature of criminal offences referred to in the sections.
2. No payment as referred to in the sections of the Act has been made to me or will be made to me or any other person.
3. I am giving the consent and authorization to remove my …………………………….. (name of organ/tissue) of my own free will without any undue pressure, inducement, influence or allurement.
4. I have been given a full explanation of the nature of the medical procedure involved and the risks involved for me in the removal of my ………………………….. (name of organ)/tissue). That explanation was given by (name of registered medical practitioner).
5. I understand the nature of that medical procedure and of the risks to me as explained by that practitioner.
6. I understand that I may withdraw my consent to the removal of that organ at any time before the operation takes place.
7. I state that particulars filled by me in the form are true and correct to the best of my knowledge and belief and nothing material has been concealed by me.

…………………………..   …......…………………………………………

                                         Date Signature of the prospective donor
                                                (Full Name)

Note: To be sworn before Notary Public, who while attesting shall ensure that the person/persons swearing the affidavit(s) signs(s) on the Notary Register, as well.

FORM 2
FOR ORGAN OR TISSUE DONATION BY LIVING SPOUSAL DONOR
(To be completed by him/her)
(Refer rules 3, 5(3)(a) and 5(3)(d))

My full name (proposed donor) is ....
....

and this is my photograph

Photograph of the Donor
(Attested by Notary Public
across the photo after affixing)

To be affixed here.

My permanent home address is ....
.... Tel: ....
My present address for correspondence is ....
.... Tel: ....
Date of birth .... (day/month/year)
I authorize removal for therapeutic purposes and consent to donate my ....
(Name of organ) to my husband/wife.................................... .... whose particulars are as
follows and full name is .... and who was born on
(Day/month/year):

Photograph of the Recipient
(Attested by Notary Public
across the photo after affixing)

To be affixed here.

I enclose copies of the following documents **(attach attested photocopy of at least two of following relevant documents to indicate the spousal relationship):**
- Ration/Consumer Card number and Date of issue and place: ....and/or
- Voter's Identity Card number, date of issue, Assembly constituency ....and/or
- Passport number and country of issue .... and/or
- Driving License number, Date of issue, licensing authority.. and/or
- Permanent Account Number (PAN) .... and/or
- AADHAAR No. (issued by Unique Identification Authority of India) ....and/or
- Any other proof of identity and address establishing spousal relationship ....
   I submit the following as evidence of being married to the recipient:-
   (a) A certified copy of a marriage certificate.
             OR
   (b) An affidavit of a 'near relative' confirming the status of marriage to be sworn before Class-I Magistrate/ Notary Public.
   (c) Family photographs.
   (d) Letter from Head of Gram Panchayat / Tehsildar / Block Development Officer/Member of Legislative Assembly/Member of Legislative Council (MLC)/Member of Parliament with seal certifying factum and status of marriage.
             OR
   (e) Other credible evidence
I solemnly affirm and declare that sections 2, 9 and 19 of the Transplantation of Human Organs Act, 1994 (42 of 1994), have been explained to me and I confirm that ....

1. I understand the nature of criminal offences referred to in the sections.
2. No payment of money or money's worth as referred to in the Sections of the Act has been made to me or will be made to me or any other person.
3. I am giving the authorisation to remove my ……………………………………………….. (organ) and consent to donate the same, of my own free will without any undue pressure, inducement, influence or allurement.
4. I have been given a full explanation of the nature of the medical procedure involved and the risks involved for me in the removal of my …………………….. (organ). That explanation was given by …………………….. (name of registered medical practitioner).
5. I understand the nature of that medical procedure and of the risks to me as explained by that practitioner.
6. I understand that I may withdraw my consent to the removal of that organ at any time before the operation takes place.
7. I state that particulars filled by me in the form are true and correct to the best of my knowledge and nothing material has been concealed by me.

…….……………………..………………………..

Date …………………….

Signature of the prospective donor
(Full Name)

Note: To be sworn before Notary Public, who while attesting shall ensure that the person/persons swearing the affidavit(s) signs(s) on the Notary Register, as well.

FORM 3
FOR ORGAN OR TISSUE DONATION BY OTHER THAN NEAR RELATIVE LIVING DONOR
(To be completed by him/her)
(Refer rules 3, 5(3)(a) and 5(3)(e))

My full name is ....
and this is my photograph

Photograph of the Donor
(Attested by Notary Public
across the photo after affixing)

| To be affixed here. |

My permanent home address is...
....Tel:...........
My present address for correspondence is ....
....Tel: ....
Date of birth .... (day/month/year)

I enclose copies of the following documents: (attach attested photocopy of at least two of following relevant documents to prove your identity):
- Ration/Consumer Card number and Date of issue and place: .... and/or
  (Photocopy attached)
- Voter's I-Card number, date of issue, Assembly constituency .... and/or
  (Photocopy attached)
- Passport number and country of issue .... and/or
  (Photocopy attached)
- Driving Licence number, Date of issue, licensing authority..................................... and/or
  (Photocopy attached)
- PAN .... and/or
- No .... and/or
- Other proof of identity and address ....

Details of last three years income and vocation of donor (enclose documentary evidence) ....
I authorize removal for therapeutic purposes and consent to donate my .... (Name of organ/tissue) to a person whose full name is .... and who was born on .... (day/month/year) and whose particulars are as follows:

Photograph of the Recipient
(Attested by Notary Public
across the Photo after affixing)

| To be affixed here. |

(attach attested photocopy of at least two relevant documents to prove identity of recipient)
- Ration/Consumer Card number and Date of issue and place: ....
  and/or
  (Photocopy attached)
- Voter's I-Card number, date of issue, Assembly constituency .... and/or
  (Photocopy attached)
- Passport number and country of issue .... and/or
  (Photocopy attached)

- Driving Licence number, Date of issue, licensing authority ……………………….......................... and/or
  (Photocopy attached)
- PAN ……………......……………………………………………………………………………………... and/or
- No ……………………….....……………………………………………………………………….…... and/or
- Other proof of identity and address ……………………………………………………….........................…

I solemnly affirm and declare that Sections 2, 9 and 19 of the Transplantation of Human Organs Act, 1994 (42 of 1994), have been explained to me and I confirm that

1. I understand the nature of criminal offences referred to in the Sections.
2. No payment of money or money's worth as referred to in the Sections of the Act has been made to me or will be made to me or any other person.
3. I am giving the consent and authorization to remove my …………………………….. (name of organ/tissue) of my own free will without any undue pressure, inducement, influence or allurement.
4. I have been given a full explanation of the nature of the medical procedure involved and the risks involved for me in the removal of my ………………………….. (name of organ/tissue). That explanation was given by ……………………………………… (name of registered medical practitioner).
5. I understand the nature of that medical procedure and of the risks to me as explained by the practitioner.
6. I understand that I may withdraw my consent to the removal of that organ at any time before the operation takes place.
7. I state that particulars filled by me in the form are true and correct to the best of my knowledge and nothing material has been concealed by me.

Date ………………………………………….   …………………………………………..

                                                        Signature of the prospective donor
                                                        (Full Name)

Note: To be sworn before Notary Public, who while attesting shall ensure that the person/persons swearing the affidavit(s) signs(s) on the Notary Register, as well.

FORM 4
FOR CERTIFICATION OF MEDICAL FITNESS OF LIVING DONOR
(To be given by the Registered Medical Practitioner)
[Refer proviso to rule 5(3)(b)]

I, Dr. ………………………………….. possessing qualification of ……………………......................... registered as medical practitioner at serial No …………………........... by the……………………. Medical Council, certify that I have examined Shri/ Smt./ Km…………………….. S/o, D/o, W/o Shri …………………… ……………………………… aged …………................................. who has given informed consent for donation of his/her …………… (Name of the organ) to Shri/Smt./Km. …………………........................... who is a 'near relative' of the donor/other than near relative of the donor and has been approved by the competent authority or Authorisation Committee (as the case may be) and it is certified that the said donor is in proper state of health, not mentally challenged * and is medically fit to be subjected to the procedure of organ or tissue removal.

Place: …………………….

………………………………………… ……

Signature of Doctor Seal

Date: ……………………..

<table>
<tr><td>

To be affixed
(pasted) here.

</td><td>

To be affixed
(pasted) here.

</td></tr>
</table>

Photograph of the Donor
(Attested by doctor)

Photograph of the recipient
(Attested by the doctor)

The signatures and seal should partially appear on photograph and document without disfiguring the face in photograph.

*In case of doubt for mentally challenged status of the donor, the Registered Medical Practitioner may get the donor examined by psychiatrist.

FORM 5

FOR CERTIFICATION OF GENETIC RELATIONSHIP OF LIVING DONOR WITH RECIPIENT

(To be filled by the head of Pathology Laboratory certifying relationship)

[Refer rules 5(3)(c) and 18(3)]

I, Dr./Mr./Mrs./Miss. ....…….……………….................….. working as …..

at ...…... and possessing qualification of …...…...................... certify that Shri/

Smt./ Km. .…... S/o, D/o, W/o Shri/Smt ....

aged …............ the donor and Shri/Smt ...….……..

S/o, D/o, W/o Shri/Smt .... aged …..….........the prospective recipient

of the organ to be donated by the said donor are related to each other as brother/sister/mother/father/son/
daughter, grandmother, grandfather, grandson and granddaughter as per their statement. The fact of this
relationship has been established / not established by the results of the tests for DNA profiling. The results of
the tests are attached.

Signature

(To be signed by the Head of the Laboratory)

Seal

Place ....

Date ....

FORM 6

FOR SPOUSAL LIVING DONOR

(To be filled by competent authority* and Authorisation Committee, of the hospital or district or state in case of foreigners)

[Refer rule 18(2)]

I, Dr./Mr./Mrs/Miss. ....…….. possessing qualification of...registered as medical practitioner at serial No .... by the .... Medical Council, certify that:

Mr. .... S/o …...................... .... aged ....

Resident of ....… and Mrs ....… D/o,W/o ....… aged …...............….....................… resident of …..….. are related to each other as spouse according to the statement given by them and their statement has been confirmed by means of following evidence before effecting the organ removal from the body of the said Shri/Smt/................................ (Applicable only in the cases where considered necessary).

OR

In case the Clinical condition of Shri/Smt …........................….. mentioned above is such that recording of his/her statement is not practicable, reliance will be placed on the documentary evidence(s).

(mention documentary evidence(s) here) ....

    (a) Marriage certificate indicate date of marriage:

    (b) Marriage photographs:

    (c) Date when transplantation was advised by the hospital (to be compared with duration of marriage):

    (d) Number and age of children and their birth certificates:

    (e) Any other document:

Signature of competent authority*/authorisation committee in case of foreigners along with Seal/Stamp

Place ....

Date ....

*Director or Medical Superintendent or In Charge of the hospital or the internal committee of the hospital formed for the purpose as, defined under the rules of Transplantation of Human Organ Act, 1994(42 of 1994).

FORM 8

FOR DECLARATION CUM CONSENT

(To be filled by near relative or lawful possessor of brain stem dead person)

[*Refer rules 5(1)(b), 5(4)(b) and 5(4)(d)*]

DECLARATION AND CONSENT FORM

I, ……………………………………… S/o, D/o, W/o. ……..…….....…………
aged ………….........................….. resident of ……………………………….......................................……….......
in the presence of persons mentioned below, hereby declare that:

1. I have been informed that my relative (specify relation) …………………………………………………………

    S/o,D/o,W/o …………………………………… aged ……………… has been declared brain stem dead / dead.

2. To the best of my knowledge (Strike off whichever is not applicable):

    (a) He/ She (Name of the deceased)... had/had not, authorised before his/her
    death, the removal of.. (Name of organ/tissue/both) of his/her body
    after his/her death for therapeutic purpose. The documentary proof of such authorisation is enclosed/
    not available.
    (b) He/ She (Name of the deceased)... had not revoked the authority as at No. 2 (a)
    above (If applicable).
    (c) There are reasons to believe that no near relative of the said deceased person has objection to any of
    his/her organs/tissue being used for therapeutic purposes.

3. I have been informed that in the absence of such authorisation, I have the option to either authorise or
    decline donation of organ/tissue/both including eye/cornea of ……………………………… (Name of the
    deceased) for therapeutic purposes. I also understand that if corneas/eyes are not found suitable for
    therapeutic purpose, then may be used for education/research.

4. I hereby authorise/do not authorize removal of his/her body organ(s) and/or tissue(s), namely (Any
    organ and tissue/Kidney/Liver/Heart/Lungs /Intestine/Cornea/Skin/Bone/Heart Valve/Any other;
    please specify) …………………………..............for therapeutic purposes. I also give permission for drawing of
    a blood sample for serology testing and am willing to share social/behavioural and medical history to
    facilitate proper screening of the donor for safe transplantation of the organs/ tissues.

Date……………………   Signature of near relative /person in lawful possession of the dead body,
and address for correspondence*

Place …………....................………… Telephone No ……………………….. Email: ……….…………………………

* in case of the minor the declaration shall be signed by one of the parent of the minor or any near relative
authorised by the parent. In case the near relative or person in lawful possession of the body refuses to sign
this form, the same shall be recorded in writing by the Registered Medical Practitioner on this Form.

(Signature of Witness 1)

1. Shri/Smt./Km ……….....………… S/o, D/o, W/o ………………………….........…………………………........

    aged …………........……….. resident of ....

    Telephone No.. Email: ....

(Signature of Witness 2)

2. Shri/Smt./Km .... S/o, D/o, W/o ....

    aged………………...........................….. resident of ………………………………………………………………….

    Telephone No .... Email: ....

FORM 9
FOR UNCLAIMED BODY IN A HOSPITAL OR PRISON
(To be completed by person in lawful possession of the unclaimed body)
[Refer rule 5(1)(b)]

I, ...S/o, D/o, W/o ....

aged.............................Resident of...having lawful possession of the dead body of

Shri/Smt./Km .... S/o, D/o, W/o .... aged....................

resident of ....and having known that no person has come forward
to claim the body of the deceased after 48 hours of death and there being no reason to believe that any person
is likely to come to claim the body I hereby, authorise removal of his/her body organ(s) and/or tissue(s),
namely..for therapeutic purposes.

Signature, Name, designation and Stamp of person in lawful possession of the dead body

Dated..............................

Place...........................

Address for correspondence ....

....

....

Telephone No ....

Email ....

(Signature of Witness 1)

1. Shri/Smt./Km .... S/o, D/o, W/o ....

   aged .... resident of ....

   Telephone No. .... Email ....
   (Signature of Witness 2)

2. Shri/Smt./Km.. S/o, D/o, W/o...

   aged .... resident of ....

   Telephone No.. Email ....

FORM 10

FOR CERTIFICATION OF BRAIN STEM DEATH

(To be filled by the board of medical experts certifying brain stem death)

[Refer rules 5(4)(c) and 5(4)(d)]

We, the following members of the Board of medical experts after careful personal examination hereby certify that Shri/Smt./Km. .... aged about .... son of/wife of/daughter of .... Resident of .... is dead on account of permanent and irreversible cessation of all functions of the brain stem. The tests carried out by us and the findings therein are recorded in the brain stem death Certificate annexed hereto.

Dated ....   Signature...................................

1. R.M.P.- Incharge of the Hospital In which brain stem death has occurred.
2. R.M.P. nominated from the panel of Names sent by the hospitals and approved by the Appropriate Authority.
3. Neurologist/Neuro-Surgeon
4. R.M.P. treating the aforesaid deceased person

(where Neurologist/Neurosurgeon is not available, any Surgeon or Physician and Anaesthetist or Intensivist, nominated by Medical Administrator In-charge from the panel of names sent by the hospital and approved by the Appropriate Authority shall be included)

BRAIN STEM DEATH CERTIFICATE

(A) PATIENT DETAILS ....

1. Name of the patient: Mr./Ms..

   S.O./D.O./W.O.   Mr./Ms ....

   Sex... Age ....

2. Home Address: ....

   ....

3. Hospital Patient Registration Number (CR No.) ....

4. Name and Address of next of kin or person responsible for the patient (if none exists, this must be specified)

   ....

5. Has the patient or next of kin agreed to any donation of organ and/or tissue?

   ....

6. Is this a Medico-legal Case? Yes .... No ....

(B) PRE-CONDITIONS:

1. **Diagnosis:** Did the patient suffer from any illness or accident that led to irreversible brain damage? Specify details ....
   ....

   Date and time of accident/onset of illness ....

   Date and onset of non-reversible coma...

2. Findings of Board of Medical Experts:

   First Medical Examination ....

   Second Medical Examination ....
   (1) The following reversible causes of coma have been excluded:
       Intoxication (Alcohol)
       Depressant Drugs

Relaxants (Neuromuscular blocking agents)
Primary hypothermia
Hypovolaemic shock
Metabolic or endocrine disorders
Tests for absence of brain stem functions

(2) Coma
(3) Cessation of spontaneous breathing
(4) Pupillary size
(5) Pupillary light reflexes
(6) Doll's head eye movements
(7) Corneal reflexes (Both sizes)
(8) Motor response in any cranial nerve distribution, any responses to stimulation of face, limb or trunk.
(9) Gag reflex
(10) Cough (Tracheal)
(11) Eye movements on caloric testing bilaterally
(12) Apnoea tests as specified
(13) Were any respiratory movements seen?
....

Date and time of first testing: ....

Date and time of second testing: ....

    This is to certify that the patient has been carefully examined twice after an interval of about six hours and on the basis of findings recorded above, Mr./Ms .... is declared brain stem dead.

Date: ....

Signatures of members of Brain Stem Death (BSD) Certifying Board as under:
  1. Medical Administrator In-charge of the hospital
  2. Authorised specialist.
  3. Neurologist/Neuro surgeon
  4. Medical Officer treating the patient.

Note:
  I. Where Neurologist/Neurosurgeon is not available, then any Surgeon or Physician and Anaesthetist or Intensivist, nominated by Medical Administrator In-charge of the hospital shall be the member of the board of medical experts for brain stem death certification.
  II. The minimum time interval between the first and second testing will be six hours in adults. In case of children 6 to 12 years of age, 1 to 5 years of age and infants, the time interval shall increase depending on the opinion of the above BSD experts.
  III. No. 2 and No. 3 will be co-opted by the Administrator In-charge of the hospital from the Panel of experts (*Nominated by the hospital and approved by the Appropriate Authority*).

FORM 11
APPLICATION FOR APPROVAL OF TRANSPLANTATION FROM LIVING DONOR
(To be completed by the proposed recipient and the proposed living donor)
[Refer rules 5(3)(d), 5(3)(e) and 10]

To be self attested across the affixed photograph without disfiguring face		To be self attested across the affixed photograph without disfiguring face
Photograph of the Donor		Photograph of the recipient

Whereas I …….......…….......…….. S/o, D/o, W/o, Shri/Smt. …………...................... aged ….......................................
residing at ……………………………………………………... have been advised by my
doctor …………….. that I am suffering from ……………………………………… and may
be benefited by transplantation of …………………………….. into my body.

And whereas I ……………………………………… S/o, D/o, W/o, Shri/Smt……......…………...
aged ……................... residing at……………………………………………………………………………...... by the
following reason(s):-

     a. by virtue of being a near relative i.e. …………………………………………............

     b. by reason of affection/attachment/other special reason as explained below:-

     ……………………………………………………………………………….....…….......................................…..

     …………………………………………………………………………………………………...........................

     I would therefore like to donate my (name of the organ) ……………………………........................ to
Shri/Smt. ………………………………...
We ………………………….. and ………………………………………….............

         (Donor)   (Recipient)

hereby apply to competent authority/Authorisation Committee for permission for such transplantation to be carried out.

     We solemnly affirm that the above decision has been taken without any undue pressure, inducement, influence or allurement and that all possible consequences and options of organ transplantation have been explained to us.

Instructions for the applicants:

1. Form 11 must be submitted along with the completed Form 1 or Form 2 or Form 3 as may be applicable.
2. The applicable Form, i.e. Form 1 or Form 2 or Form 3 as the case may be, should be accompanied with all documents mentioned in the applicable form and all relevant queries set out in the applicable form must be adequately answered.
3. Completed Form 5 must be submitted along with the laboratory report.
4. The doctor's advice recommending transplantation must be enclosed with the application.
5. In addition to above, in case the proposed transplant is between unrelated persons, appropriate evidence of vocation and income of the donor as well as the recipient for the last three years must be enclosed with this application. It is clarified that the evidence of income does not necessarily mean the proof of income-tax returns, keeping in view that the applicant(s) in a given case may not be filing income tax returns.
6. The application shall be accepted for consideration by the competent authority/Authorisation Committee only if it is complete in all respects and any omission of the documents or the information required in the forms mentioned above, shall render the application incomplete.
7. When the donor is unrelated and the donor and/or recipient belong to a State/Union Territory other than the State/Union Territory, where the transplant is intended to take place, then the Tehsildar or the officer

authorised for the purpose of the domicile state of the donor or recipient as the case may be, would provide the verification certificate of domicile of donor/recipient, as the case may be as per Form 20. The approval for transplantation would be considered by the authorisation committee of the State/District/hospital (as the case may be) where the transplantation is intended to be done. Such verification Certificate will not be required for near relatives including cases involving swapping of organs (permissible between near relatives only).

We have read and understood the above instructions.

Signature of the Prospective Donor

Signature of Prospective Recipient

....

....

Address for correspondence:

Address for correspondence:

Date:

Date:

Place:

Place:

FORM 12

APPLICATION FOR REGISTRATION OF HOSPITAL TO CARRY OUT ORGAN OR TISSUE TRANSPLANTATION OTHER THAN CORNEA
(To be filled by head of the institution)
(Refer rule 24(1))

To

The Appropriate Authority for organ transplantation ....…....................................

(State or Union territory)

We hereby apply to be registered as an institution to carry out organ/tissue transplantation.

Name(s) of organ (s) or tissue (s) for which registration is required..…..

The required data about the facilities available in the hospital are as follows:-

(A) HOSPITAL:

1. Name:
2. Location:
3. Government/Private:
4. Teaching/Non-teaching:
5. Approached by:

Road:	Yes	No
Rail:	Yes	No
Air:	Yes	No

6. Total bed strength:
7. Name of the disciplines in the hospital:
8. Annual budget:
9. Patient turn-over/year:

(B) SURGICAL FACILITIES:

1. No. of beds:
2. No. of permanent staff members with their designation:
3. No. of temporary staff with their designation:
4. No. of operations done per year.
5. Trained persons available for transplantation
   (Please specify Organ for transplantation)

(C) MEDICAL FACILITIES:

1. No. of beds:
2. No. of permanent staff members with their designation:
3. No. of temporary staff members with their designation:
4. Patient turnover per year:
5. Trained persons available for transplantation
   (Please specify Organ for transplantation):
6. No. of potential transplant candidates admitted per year:

(D) ANAESTHESIOLOGY:

1. No. of permanent staff members with their designations:
2. No. of temporary staff members with their designations:
3. Name and No. of operations performed:
4. Name and No. of equipments available:
5. Total No. of operation theatres in the hospital:
6. No. of emergency operation theatres:
7. No. of separate transplant operation theatre:

(E) I.C.U./H.D.U. FACILITIES:

1. I.C.U./H.D.U. facilities: Present............................ Not present...
2. No. of I.C.U. and H.D.U. beds:

3. Trained:-
Nurses:
Technicians:
4. Name of equipment in I.C.U.

(F) OTHER SUPPORTIVE FACILITIES:

Data about facilities available in the hospital:

(F1) LABORATORY FACILITIES:

1. No. of permanent staff with their designations:
2. No. of temporary staff with their designations:
3. Names of the investigations carried out in the Department:
4. Name and number of equipments available:

(F2) IMAGING FACILITIES:

1. No. of permanent staff with their designations:
2. No. of temporary staff with their designations:
3. Names of the investigations carried out in the Department:
4. Name and number of equipments available:

(F3) HAEMATOLOGY FACILITIES:

1. No. of permanent staff with their designations:
2. No. of temporary staff with their designations:
3. Names of the investigations carried out in the Department:
4. Name and number of equipments available:

(F4) BLOOD BANK FACILITIES (Inhouse or access): Yes .... No..

(F5) DIALYSIS FACILITIES: Yes .... No ....

(F6) Transplant coordinators (Eye Donation Counselors, in case of Cornea Transplantation):

	Yes	No
Number Posted:		
Number Trained:		

(F7) OTHER SUPPORTIVE EXPERT PERSONNEL:

1. Nephrologist   Yes/No
2. Neurologist   Yes/No
3. Neuro-Surgeon   Yes/No
4. Urologist   Yes/No
5. G.I. Surgeon   Yes/No
6. Paediatrician   Yes/No
7. Physiotherapist   Yes/No
8. Social Worker   Yes/No
9. Immunologists   Yes/No
10. Cardiologist   Yes/No
11. Respiratory physician   Yes/No
12. Others.............................   Yes/No

The above said information is true to the best of my knowledge and I have no objection to any scrutiny of our facility by authorised personnel. A Bank Draft/cheque of Rs. 10000/ (for new registration) and Rs. 5000 (for renewal) in favour of .... is enclosed.

Sd/-

HEAD OF THE INSTITUTION

FORM 13

APPLICATION FOR REGISTRATION OF HOSPITAL TO CARRY OUT ORGAN/TISSUE RETRIEVAL
OTHER THAN EYE/CORNEA RETRIEVAL
(To be filled by head of the institution)
(Refer rule 24(1))

Note: Retrieval Hospitals may also be identified based on pre-defined criteria and registered as retrieval hospital by the appropriate authority.

To

　　The Appropriate Authority for organ transplantation ....
　　(State or Union territory)
　　We hereby apply to be registered as an institution to carry out organ/tissue retrieval.

The required data about the facilities available in the hospital are as follows:-

(A)　HOSPITAL:
　　1.　Name:
　　2.　Location:
　　3.　Government/Private:
　　4.　Teaching/Non-teaching:
　　5.　Approached by:

Road:	Yes	No
Rail:	Yes	No
Air:	Yes	No

　　6.　Total bed strength:
　　7.　Name of the disciplines in the hospital:
　　8.　Annual budget:
　　9.　Patient turnover/year:

(B)　SURGICAL FACILITIES:
　　1.　No. of beds:
　　2.　No. of permanent staff members with their designation:
　　3.　No. of temporary staff with their designation:
　　4.　No. of operations done per year:
　　5.　Trained persons available for retrieval
　　　　(Please specify organ and/or tissue for retrieval):

(C)　MEDICAL FACILITIES:
　　1.　No. of beds:
　　2.　No. of permanent staff members with their designation:
　　3.　No. of temporary staff members with their designation:
　　4.　Patient turnover per year:
　　5.　Trained persons available for retrieval
　　　　(Please specify organ and/or tissue for retrieval):
　　6.　No. of critical trauma cases admitted per year.
　　7.　No. of brain stem death declared per year.

(D)　ANAESTHESIOLOGY:
　　1.　No. of permanent staff members with their designations:
　　2.　No. of temporary staff members with their designations:
　　3.　Name and No. of operations performed:
　　4.　Name and No. of equipments available:
　　5.　Total No. of operation theatres in the hospital:
　　6.　No. of emergency operation theatres:
　　7.　No. of separate retrieval operation theatre:

(E)   I.C.U./H.D.U. FACILITIES:
    1. I.C.U./H.D.U. facilities: Present............................ Not present.......................................
    2. No. of I.C.U. and H.D.U. beds:
    3. Trained:-
           Nurses:
           Technicians:
    4. Name of equipment in I.C.U.

(F)   OTHER SUPPORTIVE FACILITIES:

Data about facilities available in the hospital:

(F1)   LABORATORY FACILITIES:

    1. No. of permanent staff with their designations:
    2. No. of temporary staff with their designations:
    3. Names of the investigations carried out in the Deptt.:
    4. Name and number of equipments available:

(F2)   IMAGING FACILITIES:

    1. No. of permanent staff with their designations:
    2. No. of temporary staff with their designations:
    3. Names of the investigations carried out in the Deptt.:
    4. Name and number of equipments available:

(F3)   HAEMATOLOGY FACILITIES:

    1. No. of permanent staff with their designations:
    2. No. of temporary staff with their designations:
    3. Names of the investigations carried out in the Deptt.:
    4. Name and number of equipments available:

(F4)   BLOOD BANK FACILITIES: (in house or access)   Yes .... No....................

(F5)   Transplant coordinators: Yes .... No....................
    Number Posted:
    Number Trained

The above said information is true to the best of my knowledge and I have no objection to any scrutiny of our facility by authorised personnel. I hereby give an undertaking that we shall make the facilities of the hospital including the retrieval team of the hospital available for retrieval of the organ/tissue as and when needed.

Sd/-

HEAD OF THE INSTITUTION

FORM 14
APPLICATION FOR REGISTRATION OF TISSUE BANKS OTHER THAN EYE BANKS
(To be filled by head of the institution)
(Refer rule 24(1))

To

The Appropriate Authority for organ transplantation ....……......

(State or Union Territory)

We hereby apply to be registered as Tissue bank, Name:

Name(s) of tissue (s) (Bone, heart valves, skin, cornea, etc) for which Registration is required ....

The required data about the facilities available in the institution are as follows:-

A. General Information:
   1. Name
   2. Address
   3. Government/Private/NGO
   4. Teaching/Non-teaching
   5. Approached by:
      Rail: Yes/No
      Road: Yes/No
      Air: Yes/No
   6. Information Education and Communication (IEC) for Tissue Donation
   7. Type of tissue bank: Auto Logons/Allograph/Both

B. DONOR SCREENING REMOVAL OF TISSUE AND STORAGE:
   1. Availability of adequate trained and qualified personnel for removal tissue (annex detail)   Yes/No
   2. Names, qualification and address of the doctors/technician who will be doing removal
      of tissue. (annex details)   Yes/No
   3. Facilities for removal of Tissues   Yes/No
   4. Whether register of recipient waiting list available   Yes/No
   5. Telephone arrangement available (Telephone Number................)   Yes/No
   6. Availability of ambulance/vehicle or funds to Pay taxi for collecting tissue from outside·   Yes/No
   7. Sets of instruments for removal of tissue   Yes/No
   8. Facilities for processing of tissue   Yes/No
   9. Refrigerator for preservation of tissue   Yes/No
   10. Special containers for preservation of tissue during transit   Yes/No
   11. Suitable preservation media   Yes/No
   12. Any other specific requirement as per tissue   Yes/No

C. PRESERVATIONS OF TISSUE Arrangement of preservation of Tissue   Yes/No

D. RECORDS
   1. Arrangement for maintaining the records   Yes/No
   2. Arrangement for registration of cases, donors and follow-up of cases.   Yes/No

E. EQUIPMENT:

Instruments specific for the tissue   Yes/No

F. LABORATORY FACILITIES (If the information is exhaustive please annex it)
   (a) Names of the investigations carried out in the department
   (b) Facility for testing for: Yes/No
       i. Human Immunodeficiency Virus Type I and II
       ii. Hepatitis B Virus–HBc and HBs
       iii. Hepatitis C Virus–HCV
       iv. Syphilis–VDRL
   (c) If no where do you avail it? Please mention name and address of institute.
   (d) Facility for culture and sensitivity of tissue   Yes/No

G. OTHER PERSONNEL

1. No. of permanent staff member with their designation.
2. No. of temporary staff with their designation
3. No. of trained persons

ANY OTHER INFORMATION

The above said information is true to the best of my knowledge and I have no objection to any scrutiny of our facility by authorised personnel. A bank draft/cheque of Rs. 10000/ (for new registration) and Rs. 5000 (for renewal) in favour of .... is enclosed.

Sd/-

HEAD OF THE INSTITUTION

FORM 15
APPLICATION FOR REGISTRATION OF EYE BANK, CORNEAL TRANSPLANTATION CENTRE, EYE RETRIEVAL CENTRE UNDER TRANSPLANTATION OF HUMAN ORGANS ACT
[Refer rule 24(1)]

I. EYE BANKING:		
A.	EYE BANK and institution affiliated Ophthalmic/General Hospital 1. Name 2. Address 3. Government/Private/Voluntary 4. Teaching/Non-teaching 5. IEC for Eye Donation	
B.	REMOVAL OF EYE BALLS AND STORAGE:	
	1. Availability of adequate trained and qualified personnel for removal of whole globe or corneal (annex detail)	Yes/No
	2. Names, qualification and address of the designated staff who will be doing removal of whole globe/cornea retrieval. (annex details)	Yes/No
	3. Availability of following as per requirement: a) Whether register maintained for tissue request received from surgeon of corneal transplant centre.	Yes/No
	b) Telephone arrangement available. (Dedicated Telephone Number................)	Yes/No
	c) Transport facility for collecting Eyeballs from outside:	Yes/No
	d) Sets of instruments for removal of whole globe/cornea as per requirement	Yes/No
	e) Special bottles with stands for preservation of Eyeballs/cornea during transit.	Yes/No
	f) Suitable preservation media	Yes/No
	g) Biomedical Waste Management.	Yes/No
	h) Uninterrupted Power supply.	Yes/No
C	Manpower 1. Incharge/Director (Ophthalmologist)-1 2. Eye Bank Technician-2 3. Eye Donation Counselors (EDC)-2 per attached HCRP (Hospital Cornea Retrieval Cornea Programme) Hospital, who will be posted at eye Bank. 4. Multi-task Staff (MTS) -2	
D.	Space requirement for eye banks (400 sq ft minimum)	Yes/No
E.	RECORDS 1. Arrangement for maintaining the records	Yes/No
	2. Arrangement for registration of pledges/donors and maintenance of utilization report	Yes/No
	3. Computer with internet facility and Printer	Yes/ No
F.	EQUIPMENT: 1. Slit Lamp Biomicroscope-1 2. Specular Microscope for Eye Bank-1 3. Laminar flow (Class II)-1 4. Sterilization facility (In-house or outsourced) 5. Refrigerator with temperature monitoring for preservation of eyeballs/Cornea-1	Yes/No

G.	**LABORATORY FACILITIES**	
	1. Facility for HIV, Hepatitis B and C testing.	Yes/No
	2. If no where do you avail it? Please mention Name and address of institute.	Yes/No
	3. Facility for culture and sensitivity of Corneoscleral ring.	Yes/No
H.	**RENEWAL OF REGISTRATION:**	
	Period of renewal 5 years after last registration. Minimum of 50 corneas to be collected in 5 years. Maintenance of eye bank standards (as per Guidelines)	
II.	**EYE RETRIEVAL CENTRE (ERC):**	
A.	RETRIEVAL CENTRE—A centre affiliated to an Eye Bank 1. Name 2. Address 3. Government/Private/Voluntary 4. Teaching/Non-teaching 5. Information, Education and Communication Activities for Eye Donation 6. Name of Eye Bank to which ERC is affiliated.	
B.	**REMOVAL OF EYEBALLS AND STORAGE:**	

	1. Manpower: Adequate trained and qualified personnel for removal of eye balls/cornea (annex detail):
	  a. Incharge/Director)-1
	  b. Technician-1
	  c. MTS (Multi-task Staff)-1
	2. Transport facility (or outsource) with storage medium	

C.	Names, qualification and address of the personnel who will be doing enucleation/removal of cornea. (annex details)	
D.	AVAILABILITY OF FOLLOWING: 1. Telephone (Number ....) 2. Ambulance/vehicle or funds to pay taxi for collecting eyeballs from outside: 3. Sets of instruments for removal of eye balls/cornea 4. Special bottles with stands for preservation of 5. Eyeballs/cornea during transit: 6. Suitable preservation media 7. Waste Disposal (biomedical waste management) 8. Space requirement: Designated area	
E.	RECORDS 1. Arrangement for maintaining the records	
F.	EQUIPMENT: 1. Sterilization facility 2. Refrigerator temperature control 24 hrs for preservation of Eyeballs/Cornea. (power back up) - 1 3. The retrieval centre is affiliated with an Eye bank and Eye Bank is only authorised to distribute corneas.	
III.	**CORNEAL TRANSPLANTATION CENTRE**	
A.	1. Name of the Transplant Centre/hospital: 2. Address: 3. Government/Private/Voluntary: 4. Teaching/Non-teaching:	

		Yes/No
	5. IEC for Eye Donation: 6. Name of the registered Eye Bank for procuring tissue:	
B.	Staff details: 1. No. of permanent staff member with their designation. 2. (Note: Eye Surgeon's Experience: 3 month post MD/MS/DNB/DO) 3. No. of temporary staff with their designation 4. Trained persons for Keratoplasty and Corneal Transplantation with their names and 5. qualifications: 2 (one Corneal Transplant surgeon should be on the pay roll of the Institute)	
C.	Equipment: Slit lamp, Clinical Specular, Keratoplasty or intraocular instruments	
D.	OT facilities	
E.	Safe Storage facility	
F.	Records Registration and follow-up	
G.	Any other information	

The above said information is true to the best of my knowledge and I have no objection to any scrutiny of our facility by authorised personnel. A Bank draft/cheque of Rs. 10000/– for new registration and Rs 5000/– for renewal of registration drawn in favour of ………………………….. is enclosed.

Head of the Institute
(Name and designation)

FORM 16
CERTIFICATE OF REGISTRATION FOR PERFORMING ORGAN/TISSUE
TRANSPLANTATION/RETRIEVAL AND/OR TISSUE BANKING
[Refer rule 24(2)]

This is to certify that .... Hospital/Tissue Bank located at .... has been inspected and certificate of registration is granted for performing the organ/tissue retrieval/transplantation/ banking of the following organ(s) /tissue(s) (mention the names) under the Transplantation of Human Organs Act, 1994 (42 of 1994):

1. ....

2. ....

3. ....

4. ....

This certificate of registration is valid for a period of five years from the date of issue.

This permission is being given with the current facilities and staff shown in the present application form. Any reduction in the staff and/or facility must be brought to the notice of the undersigned.

Place ....

Signature of Appropriate Authority

Date ....

Seal: ....

FORM 17
CERTIFICATE OF RENEWAL OF REGISTRATION
(To be given by the appropriated authority on the letterhead)
[Refer rule 25(2)]

This is with reference to the application dated .... from .... (Name of the hospital/tissue bank) for renewal of certificate of registration for performing organ(s)/tissue(s) retrieval/transplantation/ banking under the Transplantation of Human Organs Act, 1994 (42 of 1994).

After having considered the facilities and standards of the above-said hospital/tissue bank, the Appropriate Authority hereby renews the certificate of registration of the said hospital/tissue bank for a period of five years.

This renewal is being given with the current facilities and staff shown in the present application form. Any reduction in the staff and/or facility must be brought to the notice of the undersigned.

Place ....

Signature of Appropriate Authority

Date ....

Seal ....

FORM 18
CERTIFICATE BY THE AUTHORISATION COMMITTEE OF HOSPITAL (IF HOSPITAL AUTHORISATION COMMITTEE IS NOT AVAILABLE THEN THE AUTHORISATION COMMITTEE OF THE DISTRICT/STATE) WHERE THE TRANSPLANTATION HAS TO TAKE PLACE
(To be issued on the letterhead)
[Refer rules 16 and 23]

This is to certify that as per application in Form 10 for transplantation of ....(Name of Organ/ tissue) from living donor, other than near relative/swap donation cases/all foreigner under the Transplantation of Human Organs Act, 1994 (42 of 1994) submitted on .... by the donor and recipient, whose details and photographs are given below, along with their identifications and verification documents, the case was considered after the personal interview of donor and recipient (if medically fit to be interviewed) and their relatives as applicable by the Authorisation Committee in the meeting held on dated ....

Details of Recipient	Details of Donor
Name..	Name:..
Age..	Age ....
Sex	Sex ....
Father/Husband Name	Father/Husband name................................
....	....
Address:	Address:..
....	....
....	....
Hospital Reg. No	Hospital Reg. No..

Relation of donor with Recipient ....

Recipient   Donor

(Photo of recipient and donor must be signed and stamped across the photo after affixing)

Permission is granted, as to the best of knowledge of the members of the committee, donation is out of love and affection and there is no financial transaction between recipient and donor and there is no pressure on/ coercion of the donor.

Permission is withheld pending submission of the following documents ....
....

Permission is not granted for the following reasons ....
....

(Member)	(Member)	(Member)
Name and Designation	Name and Designation	Name and Designation
(Member)	(Member)	(Sign of Chairman with stamp)
Health Secretary	DHS or Nominee	Name and Designation
Or Nominee	Name and Designation	

Date and place...

* In case of SWAP transplants, details are to be annexed.

FORM 19

CERTIFICATE BY COMPETENT AUTHORITY

[as defined at rule 2(c)] For Indian near relative, other than spouse, cases (In case of spousal donor, Form 6 will be applicable)

[Refer rule 5(3)(c)]

(Format for the decision of Competent Authority)

This is to certify that as per application in Form 11 for transplantation of .... (Name of Organ or Tissue) from living donor who is a near relative of the recipient under the Transplantation of Human Organs Act, 1994 (42 of 1994), submitted on .... by the donor and recipient, whose details and photographs are given below, along with their identifications and verifications documents, the case was considered after the personal interview of donor and recipient (if medically fit to be interviewed) by the competent authority in the meeting held on ....

Details of Recipient ....   Details of Donor......................................

Name...   Name:..

Age...   Age ....

Sex ....   Sex ....

Father or Husband Name ....   Father or Husband name.........................

....

Adddress: Address:

....

....

....

Hospital Reg. No ....   Hospital Reg. No...............................

Relation of donor with Recipient ....

Recipient	Donor

(Photo of recipient and donor must be signed and stamped across the photo after affixing)

Permission is granted, as to the best of knowledge of the members of the committee, donation is out of their being near relative and there is no financial transaction between recipient and donor and there is no pressure on/coercion of the donor.

Permission is withheld pending submission of following documents ....

....

Permission is not granted for the following reasons...

....

Date and place ....   (Signature and stamp of competent authority)

FORM 20
VERIFICATION CERTIFICATE IN RESPECT OF DOMICILE STATUS OF RECIPIENT OR DONOR
[To be issued by tehsildar or any other authorised officer for the purpose (required only for the donor—other than near relative or recipient if they do not belong to the state where transplant hospital identified for operation is located)]
[Refer rule 14]

PART I (To be filled by applicant donor or recipient separately in triplicate)

In reference to application for verification of domicile status for donation of ....
(Name of organ/Tissue) from living donor (other than near relative) or recipient under Transplantation of Human Organ Act, 1994 (42 of 1994), submitted on (date) .... by the applicant donor or recipient, with following details and photograph, along with his or her identification and domicile status for verification.

Details of Applicant Recipient or Donor

Name...

Age...

Sex ....

Father or Husband Name ....

....

Address:..

....

Hospital Reg. No ....

....

(Recent Photo of Applicant must be signed by him or her across the photo after affixing it)

The detail of my donor or recipient are as under and I have enclosed his or her self-signed recent photograph:

Name...

Age...

Sex ....

Father or Husband Name ....

....

Address:..

....

Hospital Reg. No ....

Signature of Applicant

Enclosure: Self-signed copy of the donor or recipient for the applicant (to be enclosed)

PART II (To be filled by the certificate issuing authority):

The above request has been examined and it is certified that the domicile status of the applicant donor or recipient mentioned as above has been verified as under:

Name .... Son or Daughter or Wife of ....

Resident of village or ward .... Tehsil or Taluka ....

District .... State or UT ....

and found correct or incorrect ....

....

Date ....

Place ....

Reference No

Authorised Signatory
Name and Designation
Office Stamp

1. The authorised signatory will handover this verification certificate to the applicant or his or her representative for submission to the Chairperson of the Authorisation Committee of the hospital or district or state (as the case may be), where transplantation has to take place.

2. The authorised signatory shall keep one copy of the above verification certificate for his records and send a copy to the Secretary, Health and Family Welfare of the State Government (Attention Appropriate authority for organ transplant) for information.

3. In case of any suspicion of organ trading, the authorised signatory mentioned above or Appropriate Authority of the state may inform police for making enquiry and taking necessary action as per the Transplantation of Human Organs Act, 1994 (42 of 1994).

FORM 21

CERTIFICATE OF RELATIONSHIP BETWEEN DONOR AND RECIPIENT IN CASE OF FOREIGNERS
(To be issued by the Embassy concerned)
[Refer rule 20(a)]

The embassy of .... (Name of Country) in India, is in receipt of an application received from
.... (Name of Organ donor and recipient) on .... (Date) recommended by
(Name of Government Department of country of origin) for facilitation of donation of .... (Name
of Organ or Tissue) from living donor .... (Name of donor) to the recipient...........................
(Name of recipient) for therapeutic purposes under the Transplantation of Human Organ Act, 1994 (42 of
1994). The details of donor and recipient and photographs are as given below:-

Details of Recipient	Details of Donor
Name..	Name:..
Age..	Age ....
Sex	Sex ....
Father or Husband Name	Father or Husband name............................
Address:	Address:..
....	....

[ ]
Recipient
[ ]
Donor

(Photo of recipient and donor must be signed and stamped across the photo after affixing)

1. This is to certify that relationship between donor and recipient is ....

2. The authenticity of following enclosed identification and verification of documents is certified

   a. ....

   b. ....

'No objection certificate' is granted, as to the best of my knowledge, the donor is donating out of love and
affection or affection and attachment towards the recipient, and there is no financial transaction between
recipient and donor and there is no pressure on or coercion of the donor.

(Signature of Senior Embassy Official)

Date:

Name: ....

Place:

Designation.......................

SOP FOR INTERSTATE ORGAN DISTRIBUTION IN BRAIN STEM DEAD (BSD) DONORS

1. Organs can only be retrieved from a Transplant Centre or Non Transplant Organ Retrieval Centre (NTORC) registered by the State Appropriate Authority.

   In case there is a potential donor in a non-registered hospital, the State Appropriate Authority of the concerned State may be requested to give the donor hospital a one-time emergency permission to carry out brain stem death (BSD) certification and organ retrieval.

   The BSD certification team must include the following:

   - The registered medical practitioner in charge of the hospital in which brain stem death has occurred;
   - An independent registered medical practitioner, being a specialist to be nominated by the registered medical practitioner in charge of the hospital in which brain stem death has occurred, from the panel of names approved by the Appropriate Authority;
   - A neurologist or a neurosurgeon to be nominated by the registered medical practitioner in charge of the hospital in which brain stem death has occurred from the panel of names approved by the Appropriate Authority; in their absence an independent registered medical practitioner, being a surgeon physician, anaesthetist or intensivist who is not a member of the transplant team, may be nominated by the registered medical practitioner in charge of the hospital in which brain stem death has occurred;
   - The registered medical practitioner treating the person whose brain stem death has occurred.

2. Organs to be donated outside the donor State must be accompanied by a letter signed by the State Appropriate Authority indicating details of the donor and the brain stem death certification, and offer of organs for distribution in another State. A sample of the required letter is attached.

3. Distribution in one State, of organs from another State, will be done as per the existing waiting lists of that State irrespective of whether there is a patient from the donor State.

4. Organs shared through ROTTO or NOTTO will be offered to States for distribution according to alphabetical order, i.e. Chhattisgarh, Dadra & Nagar Haveli, Daman & Diu, Goa, Gujarat, Madhya Pradesh, Maharashtra. Each state will be given 1 hour to respond and the offer will then move to the next State on the alphabetical list. States will be offered organs on a rotation basis.

5. In Maharashtra, organs shared through ROTTO or NOTTO will be offered to ZTCC for distribution according to alphabetical order. Each ZTCC will be given 1 hour to respond and the offer will then move to the next ZTCC on the alphabetical list. ZTCCs will be offered organs on a rotation basis.

6. Hospitals accepting organs from outside States will ensure the following:
   - send their organ retrieval team at their own cost;
   - will pay the donor Transplant Centre or Non-Transplant Organ Retrieval Centre (NTORC) for maintenance of the donor as per the existing rules laid down under the National Organ and Tissue Transplant programme (NOTP);[1] if the organs go to more than one transplant hospital payment may be recovered accordingly;
   - If the kidney or liver is donated to a government hospital then the charges for the maintenance of the deceased donor may be recovered from the government through the SOTTO of the donor hospital;
   - Will carry their own organ preservation solutions and instrument, etc.

7. If the organs are to be distributed between more than one State, then coordination will be done by ROTTO.

8. States or Union Territories that do not have transplant hospitals but who have registered NTORCs must maintain a waiting list of patients requiring organs. These patients may be registered in any transplant centre in the Region and placed on the regular waiting list of the State in which they are registered.

   However, in case of a donation from their State or Union Territory (UT) of domicile, they may be given preference as per the waiting list of their donor State or UT.

   This applies only to States and UTs that do not have registered transplant centres.

9. Each State must send ROTTO the following:
   - The name and contact details of the Appropriate Authority;
   - The name and contact details of the nodal officer who needs to be contacted during distribution of organs. The nodal officer of all States with registered transplant centres or NTORCs will be included in the ROTTO WhatsApp group for organ donation and allocation;
   - A list of all the registered transplant centres and NTORCs with the address, and the name and contact details of the registered medical practitioner in charge of the centres.
   - A copy of the State waiting list for each organ. The waiting list must also be sent to NOTTO;
   - A monthly list of all foreign nationals on the waiting lists and their current location. This waiting list must also be sent to NOTTO.
   - Post-transplant outcome of (a) recipients of BSD donors and (b) recipients of living donors, at 3 months, 6 months, 1–2 years and 5 years must be sent to ROTTO and NOTTO.
   - Post-transplant outcome of living donors at 3 months, 6 months and 1–2 years must be sent to ROTTO and NOTTO.
   - Persistent non-compliance will be addressed to NOTTO and dealt with strictly.

Dr. Astrid Lobo Gajiwala

Director, ROTTO-SOTTO, Mumbai

Protocol for Donor Information ZTCC, Pune

Following information should be provided about the donor (on WhatsApp)

Name and contact No. of Intensivist of Donor Hospital:

Time of first apnoea

Age, sex

Height and weight

Blood group

Cause of brain death, i.e. head injury, CVA

Medicolegal case   Yes/No

Date of admission to this Hospital

Date of onset of illness

Any abdominal of chest injury

Any operation on donor (nature)

Homodynamic parameters:

  Pulse, BP, Temperature, urine output

  Any episode of cardiac arrest: If yes—duration.

  Pressure support—drug and dose (current and previous)
  duration of pressure support

  Any other medications

H/O alcoholism

Viral marker status HBsAg, anti HCV

HIV

Result of latest Investigations: CBC

  ABG

Electrolytes

  Liver function: SGOT

  SGPT, S. Bilirubin (total and direct), GGT, total proteins, serum
  albumin, serum alkaline phosphatase,

Prothrombin Time, INR

  RFT = urea and creatine, urine routine, ACR BSL, HbA1c-

  USG Kidney

  USG Liver:

    Evidence of Sepsis

    2D echo or angiography simple crossmatch for heart Tx

    Lactate levels, lypase and amiles—pancreas

    CT—Thorax for Lung—Lungs Trop T (Troponin)

Glossary

Amoebiasis: Parasitic infection

Ancillary test: Supportive test

Apnoea: Stopping of breathing

Caecum: Pouch connected to junction of small/large intestine

Cytomegalovirus: Virus infection

Duodenum: First part of small intestine

Embryological: Relates to embryo/fetal development

Enterocolitis: Infection/inflammation of the large intestine

Epicardium: Inner lining of heart

Exogenous: Outside

Faeces: Stool

Fungemia: Fungal infection

GFR: Glomerular filtration rate

Haemodialysis: Method of removing waste products from blood

Hemochromatosis: Hereditary disorder whereby iron is deposited in tissues

Homeostasis: Maintain balance

Hyperoxia: Higher than normal oxygen

Ileosigmoid: Ileum = part of small intestine, sigmoid = S shaped part of large intestine

Immunoglobulins: Proteins present in blood to fight infection

Immunosuppression: To reduce the activity of the immune (defence) system

Imperceptibly transitions change that is not easily noticed

Incompatibilities: Inability to exist together

Jejunum: Middle of the small intestine

Ligaments: Tissue connecting bones to other bones or cartilage

Lymphocyte crossmatch: Blood test

Motor response: Movement of muscles

Necrotizing: Dead tissue

Orthotropic: Growing vertically

Pericardium: Sac that surrounds the heart

Peripheral neuropathy: Medical condition which affects the nerves

Peritoneal dialysis: Method to remove waste products from the blood

Pylorus: End of the stomach

Renal medulla: Part of the kidney

Serum electrolytes: Blood tests, e.g. Sodium, Potassium, chloride

Sinoatrial muscle: Present in right side of heart, regulates heart beat

Sphincter: Ring of muscle to guard an opening or tube

Valganciclovir: Antiviral medication

Septran: Antibiotic